Fundamentals of Nursing Care

A Textbook for Students of Nursing and Health Care

Books should be returned to the SDH Library on or before
the date stamped above unless a renewal has been arranged

Salisbury District Hospital Library

Fundamentals of Nursing Care

A Textbook for Students of Nursing and Health Care

Sally Hayes and Anne Llewellyn

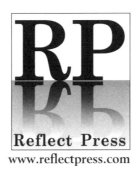

Reflect Press

www.reflectpress.com

First published in 2008

ISBN: 978 1 906052 13 3

British Library Cataloguing in Publication Data
A catalogue record for this book is available from the British Library

Production project management by Deer Park Productions

Typeset by PDQ Typesetting

Cover design by Oxmed

Printed and bound by Bell & Bain Ltd, Glasgow

Distributed by BEBC, Albion Close, Parkstone, Poole, Dorset BH12 3LL

Published by Reflect Press Ltd
11 Attwyll Avenue
Exeter
Devon, EX2 5HN
UK
01392 204400
www.reflectpress.com

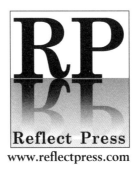

www.reflectpress.com

Contents

This book is dedicated to all of our loved ones and to all those who will, at times of both joy and suffering, be involved in caring for both them and us.

Introduction

> When I and my loved ones are sick and dying, I want our nurses to be caring, patient and tolerant – and well-educated into the bargain.
>
> (Salvage, 2001, p. 21)

A leading peer recently described nurses at a hospital in the UK as 'grubby, drunken, promiscuous, slipshod and lazy' (de Reybekill, 2008). This is a very damning picture of nurses and, hopefully, is not a perception that is widely held by the general public. Nevertheless, this high-profile quote does raise issues about the changing public perceptions of nurses and the role of the mass media in these views and opinions. What is also clear from user and carer voices and surveys of the value of nursing is that when people are ill they want health care professionals to provide competent physical care, but also emotional care. Although care and the process of caring have been a fundamental part of nursing theories and paradigms for many years, there are an increasing number of anecdotal and media stories as well as academic debates that question the extent to which this emotional caring is satisfactorily carried out, compared with the physical or technical components of nursing practice.

Since the nineteenth century, health care has developed around a positivist and scientific paradigm, with a concentration on biomedical and technological interventions and a parallel reduced focus on humanistic aspects of nursing, underpinned by the concepts of care and caring. However, recent policy initiatives – for example the *National Health Service Plan* (Department of Health (DH), 2000), *Knowledge and Skills Framework* (DH, 2004a), *Our Health, Our Care, Our Say* (DH, 2006a), Nursing and Midwifery Council *Essential Skills Clusters* (NMC, 2007) – have all emphasised the importance of patient-centred and patient-led care, quality of care and holistic principles of caring, as this introductory letter by Sir Nigel Crisp, the then Chief Executive of the NHS, demonstrates:

I strongly encourage all NHS organisations to take a close look at how they deliver their services and to ask their patients if their emotional needs are being met as well as their physical ones. They should ask patients if they are:

- getting good treatment in a comfortable, caring and safe environment, delivered in a calm and reassuring way;
- having information to make choices, to feel confident and feel in control;
- being talked to and listened to as an equal; and
- being treated with honesty, respect and dignity.

(DH, 2005a, p. iii)

User and carer surveys and anecdotal narratives have demonstrated that, although care and the humanistic aspects of nursing care are valued by the recipients of care (DH, 2002a), they are more difficult to define, quantify and therefore 'teach' to students of health care disciplines. However, as fundamental aspects of holistic nursing care in the twenty-first century, there is a need for students of nursing to not only value these aspects of nursing, but also understand their impact and relevance within the therapeutic encounter.

This book is therefore intended as a foundation level text, which focuses on fundamental principles of caring in health and social care. It is set out as a workbook, using case narratives, which are related to essential skills clusters (Nursing and Midwifery Council (NMC), 2007) to stimulate reflective learning and critical incident analysis and ground theoretical perspectives. The book can therefore be used as an independent study tool or as a core text within a particular module and in pedagogical terms will promote:

- enquiry-based learning or problem-based learning (Rideout, 2001), which is based around the concept that the starting point of learning should be a problem or a query that the individual student wishes to solve (Boud *et al.*, 1985);
- critical thinking, which is a central tenet of reflective practice (Moon, 1999);
- the exposure of tacit knowledge through reflection which promotes self-awareness and enables practitioners to evaluate their practice (Jasper,1999);
- the use of case studies and critical incident analysis as tools for reflective thinking, thus developing the ability of students to deconstruct practice and examine how to further develop competencies;
- an understanding of Carper's *Fundamental Patterns of Knowing*, which describe the various kinds of knowing about practice – these include empirical and aesthetic areas of knowledge, as well as tacit elements

and recognition of the personal meaning that underpins learning and knowledge for each individual (Carper, 1978).

The contents of this book

Chapter 1 introduces the themes and definitions of the book, asking the question 'what is the nature of nursing within its historical context?'. Frameworks for understanding nursing and learning (for example, Gibbs' reflective cycle and critical incident analysis) are introduced as well as the NMC *Essential Skills Clusters* (NMC, 2007), the *Knowledge and Skills Framework* (DH, 2004a) and *Essence of Care Benchmarks* (DH, 2001a), which essentially set the professional and policy context. Chapter 2 goes on to introduce definitions of care and the nature of caring, exploring the elements and process of caring and attributes of the carer. The relationship between caring and nursing models is explored, as well as the context of caring within the therapeutic relationship. Finally the question of whether care can be measured, and therefore quality assured, is addressed.

Chapters 3 to 7 are case studies worked around the five pathways that were identified following a series of national and regional stakeholder events in 2006, led by the Chief Nursing Officer (CNO) and taking forward recommendations set out by the CNO in *Modernising Nursing Careers: Setting the Direction* (DH, 2006c). These pathways represent those most commonly followed by patients and service users in their journey through health care services. They are:

- children, family and public health;
- first contact, access and urgent care;
- supporting long-term care;
- acute and critical care;
- mental health and psychosocial care.

Within the case studies you are asked to use reflective practice and critical incident analysis to examine the examples of care explored in the experiences of five care recipients and, where relevant, their families. You are challenged to consider the elements of nursing actions or interventions that make up the caring process, those that are important to the care recipient and to reflect on the use of 'caring interventions' such as touch, kindness, empathy, and communication. Issues such as lay professional conflict, the importance of user articulation, the concept of self and cultural competency are all considered.

Chapter 8 then goes on to explore the context of caring in the twenty-first century and the challenges that nurses may encounter in delivering humanistic elements of care in a bureaucratic health care environment that is focused on performance indicators, cost containment and efficiency.

Throughout the text links are made to the NMC *Essential Skills Clusters* (NMC, 2007) (Appendix 1) (referred to as **ESC**); The NHS *Knowledge and Skills Framework* (2004a) (Appendix 2) (referred to as **KSF**); and *The Essence of Care: Patient-focused Benchmarking for Health Care Practitioners* (DH, 2001a) (Appendix 3) (referred to as **Essence of Care**) which together set the framework for the implementation of high standards of care for nursing practitioners.

The case studies throughout the book are fictional, although some elements of them may be derived from real situations. The biographical data and details of locations are all fictional and any resemblance to reality is accidental and coincidental.

Chapter 1

Nursing Care in the Historical and Contemporary Context

> **The key issues that will be addressed in this chapter are:**
> - the contemporary policy drivers in health care;
> - an introduction to the concept of care;
> - the historical development of nursing as both a science and an art;
> - fundamental patterns of nursing knowledge, using Carper's (1978) framework of analysis;
> - reflective practice as a tool for developing nursing knowledge and its application to practice.
>
> By the end of this chapter you should be able to:
> - identify important developments in health policy that impact on contemporary nursing care;
> - explain the historical development of nursing as both a science and an art;
> - demonstrate an understanding of the nature/nurture debate in relation to gendered roles in health care practice;
> - describe Carper's fundamental patterns of knowing (1978) and understand them in the context of nursing;
> - understand the principles of reflective learning and critical incident analysis.

INTRODUCTION

While there are many examples of service users and carers experiencing good nursing care and evaluating the outcomes of nursing practice and nurse/patient relationships in a positive way, there are also a number of anecdotal stories and research findings identifying patient dissatisfactions with care and the caring relationship.

> Mrs G, 64, claimed her husband 72, was left unwashed, without drink and in pain from unbandaged burns at ————. She said the quality of nursing in his final three days was 'pathetic'. She became so concerned by his neglect at the hospital that she drew up a rota

with her daughter to make sure one of them was always at his bedside.

'I was appalled and disgusted that nurses could be just so pathetic', she said. 'I did not see any caring at all. The saddest thing for me was that on the day he died he put his arms out and said "get me out of here, take me home".'

(BBC News, 28 November 2007)

A report by the Health Care Commission (HCC) in 2007 found that some hospitals are still failing to treat people with dignity and respect (**ESC Standard 3. iv; Essence of Care: Privacy and Dignity Benchmark**), and reported incidences of people being left unwashed, without clean bed linen and wearing ill-fitting hospital gowns. Another report for the Commission for Social Care Inspection in 2007 identified poor treatment of older people in some care homes while, also in 2007, the Healthcare Commission identified deficits in the care of many people with learning difficulties.

The aim of this book is to revisit the concept of care and the process of how to care and how to enable individuals to feel cared for within the clinical encounter.

CONTEMPORARY POLICY DRIVERS

There is no doubt that the concept of care and good quality of care is central to the reforms in health care that have been introduced under New Labour since 1997. The programme of modernisation extends to all public services, and focuses on democratisation of services and emphasis on effective and efficient services. There are six broad principles for the modernisation of health care, two of which explicitly identify the need for a caring service:

- improve efficiency so that every pound in the NHS is spent to maximise the care for patients;
- shift the focus on to quality of care so that excellence is guaranteed to all patients.

(DH, 1997)

This emphasis on care and a caring service is further developed in the NHS Plan (2000) which identifies the need to 'get the basics right', refocusing the service to improve the patient/service user experience. Further to this, *The Essence of Care* (DH, 2001a) was launched in 2001 by the Modernisation Agency of the NHS with the aim of establishing benchmarks for clinical governance to help health care practitioners to adopt a patient-focused and structured approach to sharing and comparing practice.

Health care practitioners have worked with care recipients to identify best practice and to develop plans for improving quality of care, relevant to all health and social care settings. The benchmarks are therefore presented in generic format, so that they can be used in primary, secondary or tertiary care settings and with a range of user and carer groups. Initially eight benchmarks were established, but further benchmarks were added later in response to feedback from practitioners and service users. The notion of person-centred care is central to the benchmarks, with an emphasis on the promotion of self-care, respect for individual needs and preferences in the care process and the provision of high quality care.

> Patients benefit from care that is focused upon respect for the individual.
>
> (Benchmark for Privacy and Dignity, DH, 2001a)

The *Essence of Care* Benchmarks
Benchmarks have been published on:
- continence and bladder and bowel care;
- personal and oral hygiene;
- food and nutrition;
- pressure ulcers;
- privacy and dignity;
- record-keeping;
- safety of clients with mental health needs in acute mental health and general hospital settings;
- principles of self care;
- promoting health (added in 2006);
- care environment (added in 2007).

(DH, 2001a, 2006d and 2007a)

PROFESSIONAL STANDARDS FOR NURSING CARE

In 2002, the Nursing and Midwifery Council (NMC) replaced the United Kingdom Central Council (UKCC) as the body charged with establishing and maintaining a register of nurses and midwives who may legally practice, and for setting standards for the assessment and establishment of professional competency and proficiency. In 2004, the NMC established a range of competencies that nurses need to achieve in order to be admitted to the register, as determined by the context of their practice area. Thus:

'Applicants for entry to the nurses' part of the register must achieve the standards of proficiency in the practice of adult nursing, mental health nursing, learning disabilities nursing or children's nursing' (NMC, 2004).

There are 17 standards of proficiency, which nurses must demonstrate that they have achieved in order to be entered onto Level 1 of the register and therefore become eligible to practise. These standards are focused on the assessment, planning and implementation of nursing care within ethical, legal and policy frameworks and are related to the *Standards of Conduct, Performance and Ethics for Nurses and Midwives* (NMC, 2008). Throughout these standards, the concept of care either implicitly or explicitly underpins the objectives:

> The people in your care must be able to trust you with their health and wellbeing. To justify that trust, you must
> - make the care of people your first concern, treating them as individuals and respecting their dignity
> - work with others to protect and promote the health and wellbeing of those in your care, their families and carers, and the wider community
> - provide a high standard of practice and care at all times
> - be open and honest, act with integrity and uphold the reputation of your profession.
>
> (NMC, 2008)

In addition, in 2007, the NMC produced the *Essential Skill Clusters for Pre-registration Nursing Programmes*, which established standards of proficiency required for entry to branch programmes and at the point of entry to the register. These clusters relate to the provision of care, but focus on more specific achievement of learning outcomes in relation to:

- care, compassion and communication;
- organisational aspects of care;
- infection prevention and control;
- nutrition and fluid management;
- medicines management.

There is also an emphasis on nurses being able to provide care to diverse groups of care recipients, respecting cultural diversity, individual choice and dignity. In line with the government's modernisation agenda and a changing health care environment, there is a focus on the concepts of facilitating and enabling self-care and promoting health and well-being. This is also exemplified through the Scottish strategy for nursing, midwifery and allied health professionals (AHPs), *Delivering Care, Enabling Health*, which emphasises the caring role of nursing within the context of a preventative and anticipatory care service (available at **www.scot land.gov.uk**). In the words of the Chief Nursing Officer for Scotland, Paul Martin, the strategy is:

> . . . about taking traditional values forward and applying them in a modern context. That is why it was vital that we did not lose sight of the reason nurses, midwives and AHPs are here – to care for, enable, support and comfort the people who use our services.
>
> (Scottish Executive, 2006)

THE CONCEPT OF CARE

The concept of care is frequently used in relation to human relationships, nursing practice and health policy. Indeed, the term 'health care' is used to denote the organisation and delivery of services, which are provided in relation to health and illness. At some time in our lives we all give and receive care. Right through life, to varying degrees, we rely on being cared for by others or are relied on to care for others.

Activity

Draw a map of your own personal biography (e.g. being born, child-hood, going to school, friendships, first romantic relationship, etc.). Identify phases when you were a care recipient and/or a care giver.

But what do we mean by the concept of care and why is it fundamental to nursing practice? Caring takes place within the context of a relationship and involves the provision of physical, emotional and or social support by one person for another. Baines *et al.* (1991, p.11) define caring as 'The mental, emotional and physical effort involved in looking after, respond-ing to and supporting others'. Sturdy (2008) adds another dimension to the definition of caring, seeing dignity and respect for the value of a person and their right to equality as a core aspect of the caring role.

Activity

Think about a situation when you felt cared about by another person.
• Reflect on the reasons why you felt cared about.
• What attributes did the carer demonstrate?

Although various authors who discuss the concept of care will emphasise different components of the caring process, the following summary by

Watson encapsulates the core elements of care. Factors integral to the caring process include:

- cultivation of sensitivity to self and others;
- development of a helping-trusting relationship;
- promotion of acceptance of positive and negative feelings;
- provision for a supportive, protective and corrective mental, physical, socio-cultural and spiritual environment;
- assistance with the human needs of gratification.

(Watson, 1985, pp. 9–10)

Thus it can be seen that caring is a multi-faceted activity, which is experienced between at least two people. To illustrate this multifaceted nature of caring, let us imagine a clinical scenario where, as a nurse, you are required to give an injection to a care recipient (**ESC 38.ii; 38.iii**). In selecting the appropriate site, effectively cleaning the site and ensuring that the injection is given accurately, you are providing good physical care. In addition, by providing explanations of what you are doing and why, addressing and allaying any anxieties that the recipient might be experiencing, you are using communication effectively to provide cognitive and emotional care. A nurse providing good care in this scenario would also be sensitive to the care recipient's dignity, ensuring that screens or curtains were used (whether in the institutional or domestic setting) to ensure privacy. Furthermore, s/he would be sensitive to the fact that the physical task might involve touch in an area that the care recipient finds uncomfortable or intrusive and the nurse would be sensitive to the impact of this (see Chapter 7).

Morse *et al.* (1990) argue that caring is essential to human existence and is central to nursing, and nurses would no doubt claim they are caring persons (Ousey and Johnson, 2007).

> Care is the essence of nursing and the central, dominant and unifying focus of nursing.
>
> (Leininger, 1991, p. 35)

There is no single definition of nursing, but many theorists view the caring and interpersonal focus of the nurse–patient relationship as a unique feature of the role (Benner and Wrubel, 1989; Watson, 1985; Swanson, 1993).

> The focus of nursing is on the care of human beings. . .Nursing is concerned with human beings interacting with their environment in ways that lead to self-fulfillment and maintenance of health.
>
> (King, 1981, cited in Lindberg *et al.*, 1990, p. 9)

THE HISTORICAL DEVELOPMENT OF NURSING

Nursing activity has always been a feature of human societies, providing care to individuals in times of sickness. Traditionally care of the sick would take place within the family (usually by women) using remedies that had been handed down through the generations. However, nursing as an activity outside the family setting has its historical roots in religious contexts and practices, where nursing care was provided to the sick who took refuge in religious institutions by those who had taken holy orders (Peacock and Nolan, 2000).

Industrialisation in the eighteenth century led to a reduction in the significance of religious organisations and the growth of new forms of institutions. Of particular significance to nursing were the development of the workhouse system and voluntary hospitals. The workhouse system was established under the 1834 Poor Law Amendment Act, which was designed to deter pauperism. Poverty at this time was seen to be predominantly related to individual moral deficiency, whereby individuals were considered to be idle and reluctant to work or squandering their resources. The solution to this perceived problem of pauperism was to establish a deterrent system of workhouses, where conditions would be worse than the conditions of those who were able to provide for themselves. However, the assumptions about the causes of poverty failed to account for the fact that a significant number of people were unable to maintain themselves through work due to sickness. As a result of this, the workhouse was populated by large numbers of sick people, necessitating the establishment of wards to care for them. Able-bodied and healthier inmates (women) delivered nursing care within these workhouse wards, tending the sick and following a medical practitioner's instructions. There was little emphasis on care or the quality of care provision, with the primary aim of nursing being focused on physical activities.

At the same time, developments in medical knowledge in the nineteenth century led to the need for a system of hospitals to investigate and treat sick people and this resulted in the development of voluntary hospitals, which were largely funded through charitable organisations or wealthy individuals. Unqualified women would assist doctors within these hospitals and would provide care for the sick. Similarly, unqualified women might provide some sort of care for the sick and dying for some sort of payment within private homes (as illustrated by the fictional character Sairey Gamp in Charles Dickens' novel, *Martin Chuzzlewit*; Sairey Gamp was an unpleasant gin-soaked woman, whose role was to sit with the dying and lay out corpses).

Thus, before the mid-nineteenth century, nursing care was delivered by a range of unqualified and uneducated individuals (mainly women). However, in the latter part of the nineteenth century, concerns about standards of care and the need for a more regulated and educated nursing workforce led to the establishment of nursing as a distinct occupation. Florence Nightingale was highly influential in the development of training courses for nurses and the establishment of a core set of values and principles. Nightingale's emphasis was on the need for nurses to display good moral character, obedience and appropriate behaviour, and this is embodied in the Nightingale pledge that nurses were expected to take:

> I solemnly pledge myself before God and in the presence of this assembly to pass my life in purity and to practice my profession faithfully. I will abstain from what is deleterious and mischievous, and will not take or knowingly administer any harmful drug. I will do all in my power to elevate the standard of my profession, and will hold in confidence all personal matters committed to my keeping, and all family affairs coming to my knowledge in the practice of my calling. With loyalty will I endeavor to aid the physician in his work, and devote myself to the welfare of those committed to my care.
>
> (Attributed to Lystra Gretta, 1893)

Nightingale emphasised the virtues of obedience and the nurse's role in assisting the doctor, and she saw nursing as a female vocation, based on the ideals of female virtues of caring. Thus caring was seen as an innate characteristic of women, with great emphasis on the development of these characteristics in order that nursing be viewed as a legitimate and respectable occupation, in contrast to the rather tarnished image of carers such as the Sairey Gamp character. Student nurses were judged on the basis of trustworthiness, honesty, sobriety, truthfulness, quietness and neatness (Smith, 1982). Nurses were trained in relation to tasks where they could assist doctors without usurping the doctor's authority or position, leading to a gendered division of labour, with a division between the art of nursing, focused on care, and the science of medicine, with its curative focus.

Activity

- How relevant is the Nightingale pledge for contemporary nursing?
- In what ways has the profession of nursing changed since the nineteenth century?

Throughout the twentieth century, the nature of nursing has developed from this original emphasis on the virtuous and obedient woman, with many authors (Gerrish *et al.*, 2003) arguing that nursing has gone through a professionalisation strategy through the development of a body of theoretical knowledge. Initially, the focus was on the development of scientific knowledge to inform nursing practice, which continued the subservience of nursing to medicine.

> The early science of nursing was not a separate and recognised discipline, like chemistry or psychology. Instead, it was a loosely defined body of scientific facts and principles underlying physician-prescribed nursing.
>
> (Lindberg *et al.*, 1990, p. 29)

However, as an occupation subservient to medicine, nursing could not be seen as a profession in its own right, but the move of nurse education into universities (initially in the United States) led to developments in a body of distinct nursing knowledge that distinguished it from medicine. The single most important factor that distinguished this body of nursing knowledge was through the emphasis on the science of caring. A number of nursing theories and models developed, either focusing on behavioural systems (Johnson, 1980; Roy, 1980) or on nursing as an holistic science (Rogers, 1967), while Watson theorised nursing as an humanistic science with caring as a unifying concept (Watson, 1985).

NURSING AS AN ART

There has also been increased emphasis on nursing as an art, emphasising the role of caring. The art of nursing is creative in that it requires the ability to envision valid ways of helping in relation to results which are appropriate (Orem, 1980). Nursing care is determined by the way a nurse is able to use knowledge and skills to appreciate the uniqueness of the care recipient and physically and emotionally assist him/her on the merits of their particular circumstances (Stockdale and Warelow, 2000). Nursing care requires internal qualities such as personal values to be combined with nursing competencies including technical and cognitive skills (Shiber and Larson, 1991). Nursing skills encompass psychomotor acts, cognitive abilities (reasoning, communication) and phenomenological abilities (intuitiveness and knowledge based on experience) (Webber, 2002).

Nursing could be described from a caring science perspective, where individuals are viewed as unique, creative, moral and caring people. This has implications for caring, in that a moral and value dimension is added to the caring role, where each individual has a unique value base, related to a cultural and, sometimes, a religious context. Thus carers need to be aware of the individual's cultural and value base in order to treat them with respect and to acknowledge the equal value of everybody (Leininger, 1995).

Nursing theories and many nursing models identify the interpersonal nature of nursing and the emphasis on each person as a unique biological, psychological and social individual. Thus the contemporary paradigm of nursing views care as holistic, seeing individuals not just as biological beings, but operating from a bio-psychosocial stance. Theories from biological sciences, psychology and the social sciences are all relevant in informing good nursing practice.

Activity

Imagine that you are joining a dating agency or friendship club.
• Write a few lines, describing yourself to potential partners/friends.
• Reflect on how the description reflects the biological, psychological and social elements and cultural diversity of personhood.

Although there has been a development of this unique body of nursing knowledge, there remains a gendered division within the health care division of labour, with medicine being seen as based on masculine traits and nursing on feminine traits (Allen and Hughes, 2002). The notion that caring is an innate female quality is central to these gendered ideas of the nurse's caring role. However, the degree to which gender differences are innate or socialised has been the subject of much debate (the nature/nurture debate). This debate has focused on whether the differences between men's and women's behaviour are actual differences or normative differences, i.e., the way in which men and women are expected to behave. Biological explanations of gender difference focus on the fact that males and females behave differently because they have different genetic composition and biological make-up, with beliefs that males are naturally more aggressive than females, who are naturally more passive and caring.

Sociologists have drawn attention to the role of nurture and socialisation in the construction of masculinity and femininity, leading to a social construction of gendered characteristics. The family and education systems serve as institutions for the primary socialisation of children, providing the environmental and social context for the development of normative gendered traits (Macionis and Plummer, 2005). Thus boys may be encouraged not to display emotion ('big boys don't cry'), to develop practical skills and to stand up for themselves. Girls on the other hand may be encouraged to be more emotionally expressive and passive. This socialisation may be either a deliberate manipulation of behaviour, or may be done unconsciously, the stereotypical behaviours being so firmly entrenched. However, the traits associated with females are less valued in society, where there is emphasis on scientific rationality and the male breadwinner model of the labour market persists (Dex, 1980; Lewis, 1998).

> Traindrivers earn, on average, £10,000 a year more than nurses. Gender differences between the professions suggest that sexism may be the reason for the salary gap.
>
> (Waters, 2008, p.19)

Activity

When watching commercial television, take note of the adverts.
- In what ways do they portray sterotypical gendered traits?

Nurses in contemporary society are faced with a dilemma, in that nursing is practised within a society that undervalues caring, which is seen as part of the essentially passive nature of women that is either innate or socialised (Daley *et al.*, 2002). Feminists have highlighted this (Dalley, 1988; Finch and Groves, 1983), identifying the relationship between women's work and caring work. Sex-role stereotyping and the construction of gendered roles are significant in an analysis of caring. Graham (1983) argues that in order to understand the ideas that underpin caring and the gendered nature of caring, we need to distinguish between 'caring about' and 'caring for'. Caring for is concerned with performing the tasks of tending to someone's needs, while caring about is concerned with emotional attachment. Both men and women are capable of both types of care, but Dalley (1988) argues that caring about and caring for coalesce in motherhood, which is seen as an integral part of women's nature and role (see Figure 1).

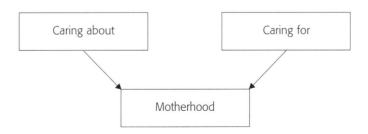

Figure 1 Caring about and caring for

However, while caring may be undervalued generally in society, at an individual level, caring and compassion are very much valued and, in particular, in the nurse/care recipient relationship. In a study in 2006, Rush and Cook identified characteristics that service users valued in nurses, including:

- good communication;
- respect;
- appropriate appearance;
- attention to hygiene;
- detailed knowledge of patients' conditions and treatments.

This was further highlighted by Carr (2000), who argued that service users very often valued the small things that nurses did for them and positively evaluated the comfort that they derived from these acts of kindness.

> Equally, small creature comforts and acts of kindness were dispro-portionately therapeutic. The kindness of the nurse who took the time to search through bags of dirty bed linen for my son's favour-ite soft toy that had been accidentally removed with a vomit-stained sheet . . .
>
> (Carr, 2000, p. 31)

It is also very strongly supported in the literature that good nurse caring results in increased health and healing and can result in a sense of solidar-ity, security, increased self-esteem, increased reality orientation, personal growth and lessening of fear and anxiety for care recipients (Brilowski and Wendler, 2005).

So how can caring be developed? While not wanting to adhere to gendered stereotypes, we do believe that socialisation is important in relation to caring and the process of caring, and that nurse education has an important role to play in the development of professional nurses who are fit for practice in the twenty-first century, and that an understanding of the nature of nursing knowledge is central to this process.

CARPER'S *FUNDAMENTAL PATTERNS OF KNOWING IN NURSING*

Carper (1978) argues that it is important to understand the knowledge that underpins an activity so that we can understand the way that that knowledge is organised and applied in practice. She identifies four patterns of knowing that underpin contemporary nursing practice. These four dimensions do not stand alone, but are integrated in the holistic approach to care and therapeutic relationships, as demonstrated in Figure 2.

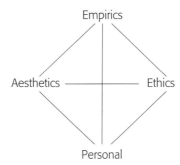

Figure 2 Diagrammatic representation of Carper's (1978) fundamental patterns of knowing in nursing

Empirics (the science of nursing)

This is factual knowledge that involves describing, explaining and predicting phenomena and answers the question – what is this?

Aesthetics (the art of nursing)

This is expressive knowledge as opposed to observable or descriptive knowledge and involves a subjective element and a direct feeling about an experience. The aesthetic of nursing involves, therefore, not just the observation and description of a care recipient's behaviour and actions, but also an understanding of their view of what is significant in terms of needs and wants and experiences. Empathy is an important concept in relation to the aesthetics of nursing, where the nurse is able to understand and appreciate the impact of an experience on another. However, this does not mean that the nurse has to have had the same experience as the care recipient (even if they had, the way that they experienced a particular situation may be different, depending on various contextual and individual factors). Empathy therefore combines knowledge with understanding of the subjective experience and application of skills and knowledge to the situation.

Ethics (the moral content of nursing knowledge)

Within the context of contemporary health care, nurses are increasingly faced with the need to make decisions and choices, and these choices raise questions about what is morally right or wrong. There is a moral code, which underpins nursing practice, based on 'the primary principle of obligation embodied in the concepts of service to people and respect for human life' (Carper, 1978, p.17). In ambiguous situations, it may be difficult to predict the consequences of one's actions and the moral content of nursing knowledge entails the making of difficult personal choices, determining what is good and bad or what ought to be done in a situation. In addition, there may be conflicts in the delivery of health and nursing care, and the ethical dimension of knowing helps to understand and resolve some of these dilemmas. For example, how does a busy nurse make a choice between the time to be allocated to the care needs and wants of different care recipients when there is limited time available? Rather than prescribing what should be done in given situations, ethical nursing knowledge provides the nurse with knowledge and insights into alternative courses of action with emphasis on the rights and dignity of the care recipient. Advocacy may be an important aspect of ethical nursing practice, where the nurse acts in a way that promotes the rights and interests of others (Mallik, 1997).

Personal knowledge (knowledge of self)

Personal knowledge involves the knowing of self and awareness of experiences based on one's own personal life knowledge. As a human activity, based on interpersonal and therapeutic relationships, personal knowledge is fundamental to good nursing practice, as this will impact on the nature and quality of the interpersonal relationships.

> ...there is growing evidence that the quality of interpersonal contacts has an influence on a person's becoming ill, coping with illness and becoming well.
>
> (Mitchell, 1973, cited in Carper, 1978)

Personal knowledge is thus concerned with an introspective awareness that allows the nurse to engage in the world of the care recipient, rather than being objectively detached from it, and to 'express an authentic, genuine self in interactions with others' (Freshwater, 2002).

> The following morning a nurse came to change the dressing on my neck. She asked if I would like to see the wound so that I would know exactly what had been done. I was struck by her thoughtfulness and the trouble she took to find a mirror for me to use.
>
> When she had finished sorting me out she asked if there was anything else I wanted. Without thinking I replied, 'I would love a hug'. I don't normally feel comfortable hugging strangers but I was used to a family life that involved a lot of physical contact, and

know enough about psychology to be aware of its importance in the wellbeing of all primates, including us.

I was feeling vulnerable, my neck hurt and I needed 'grooming'. To my delight she sat on the bed, threw open her arms and said, 'I will give you a cuddle,' and proceeded to do just that for several minutes. I can honestly say that it did me more good than the painkillers. I could feel myself relaxing, becoming more calm and genuinely feeling so much better.

(Holland, 2004)

Activity

Think about how you would react in this situation.
• What factors might influence your actions or decisions?
• How would you feel if someone with scabies and head lice asked you for a hug?

PROFESSIONAL NURSING AND CRITICAL THINKING

Nursing is a profession that operates within a dynamic health care environment and, as such, nurses are constantly learning, using a variety of learning strategies to develop theoretical and practical knowledge and to integrate the two. The Essential Skills Clusters (NMC, 2007) emphasise the importance of lifelong learning in relation to autonomous and reflective practitioners of health care. Standard 12.iii. states that nurses should be able to:

Use[s] supervision and other forms of reflective learning to make effective use of feedback.

In the past few years, there has been growing interest in reflection and reflective practice as processes of learning in health and social care (Gould, 2004). From a sociological viewpoint, this can be contextualised within a wider framework of social change. Giddens (1991) argues that we live in a pluralist and fragmented society, and there is no universal way of explaining the social world that we inhabit. There are no universal truths, but an ever-changing set of truths and individual interpretations. He goes on to say that individuals constantly interpret the social world in relation to their own personal experiences and interactions, and construct meanings about their social world through constant self-reflection on actions and interactions within the social world – he terms this 'self-reflexivity'.

15

Over the last two decades, the importance of reflection and reflective practice has been increasingly utilised as a teaching and learning strategy in nursing (Gould, 2004; Johns, 2002; Heath, 1998; Burnard, 1995), as there has been a growing acknowledgement that nursing knowledge is not only gained and developed through empirically testable facts, but also through knowledge gained through experience (experiential knowledge).

> Reflection is a means of surfacing experiential knowledge, and students may begin to use reflection as their experience of nursing accumulates.
>
> (Heath, 1998, p. 1054)

Reflection in nursing

Reflection involves looking back on an event or experience, to make sense of it and make changes where appropriate (Taylor, 2000). It is:

> ...the process of internally examining and exploring an issue of concern, triggered by an experience, which creates and clarifies meaning in terms of self, and which results in a changed conceptual perspective.
>
> (Boyd and Fales, 1983, p.100)

Activity

Think about a social situation that did not go quite as well as you had hoped.
- How did you feel about this?
- What knowledge did you use to evaluate why it had not gone as planned?
- What would you do differently if you were in a similar situation?

The concept of learning from experience is not new. In 1933 Dewey argued that people begin to reflect when there is a problem to be solved. However, the current focus on reflective practice can be traced back to the work of Schön (1983), who identified two aspects of reflection: 'reflection on action' and 'reflection in action'. Reflection on action involves thinking about something that has already been done, starting with a description of events and then moving on to a deeper examination of what happened, involving who, what, why, where sort of questions. This entails much more than just remembering or recounting a situation and is concerned with using experience to develop knowledge.

The second type of reflection, reflection in action, involves thinking about something as you are doing it, getting a feel for a situation and reflecting on alternative courses of action. This type of reflection is more likely to be used by more experienced practitioners (Benner's (1984) notion of the expert nurse, who uses intuition and experience to formulate and deliver care). The first approach to reflective learning will be used throughout this book, where case studies will be presented as learning experiences and the reader will be guided to reflect on the material and apply knowledge in order to develop understanding.

Reflection in nursing is an important aspect in bridging the theory/practice divide and analysing decisions that are made in providing care. Argyris and Schön (1974) use the term 'theory in use' to identify the way in which theory may impact on clinical decision-making. Decisions in nursing are often made in the context of a particular situation, with due consideration for the desired outcomes of actions. In practice, nurses may make decisions using their repertoire of knowledge, including experience, education, values, beliefs and past strategies (the four patterns of nursing knowledge as identified by Carper, 1978). However, the nature of nursing knowledge that is used is often implicit, and may only be made explicit through a process of critical reflection (Rich and Parker, 1995).

Reflection can occur in many different ways, depending on purpose and context. Taylor (2000) identifies three broad types of reflection:

- Technical reflection, which is based on the scientific method of developing learning, and involves rational thinking and deductive reasoning. This reflects Carper's empirical pattern of nursing knowledge.
- Practical reflection, involving description and explanation of human behaviour and which therefore has a subjective and personal element. The more self-reflexive a nurse is, the more likely they are to value emotional connections with patients (Henderson, 1991). This reflects Carper's aesthetic pattern of nursing knowledge.
- Emancipatory reflection, which is expressly linked with transformative education. The purpose of transformative education is to challenge assumptions and beliefs, leading to a change in behaviour or attitude. 'Reflection may be a vehicle through which values or beliefs can be challenged or changed' (Green, 2002, p. 5). In this way, emancipatory reflection can be liberating as practitioners are freed from assumptions or beliefs that may lead to oppressive actions. This reflects Carper's personal pattern of nursing knowledge.

Moon (2004) identifies a number of potential outcomes as a result of the process of reflection:

- learning, knowledge and understanding;
- some form of action;
- a process of critical review;
- personal and continual professional development;
- reflection on the process of learning or personal functioning (meta-cognition);
- the building of theory from observations in practice situations;
- the making of decisions/resolution of uncertainty, the solving of problems, empowerment and emancipation;
- unexpected outcomes (for example, images, ideas that could be solutions to dilemmas or seen as creative activity);
- emotion (that can be an outcome or part of the process);
- clarification and the recognition that there is need for further reflection.

(Moon, 2004, p. 84)

There are many models of reflection and reflective practice in nursing and other professional fields, but there is a general consensus that the process of reflection starts with a feeling or thought about something that happened and involves a cyclical process of analysing the event and drawing conclusions and future plans. Reflection is therefore a process that requires the use of knowledge and understanding that we already have, in order to make sense of ideas or solutions where there is not necessarily an obvious solution (Moon, 2004). Gibbs' reflective cycle (see Figure 3) clearly demonstrates the cyclical and continual process of reflection and will be utilised as the reflective model within this book.

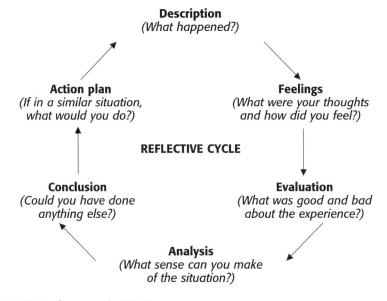

Figure 3 Gibbs' reflective cycle (1988)

Reflecting over nursing actions involves considering and analysing the experience of clinical situations. This can be achieved in a number of ways, including keeping reflective journals or diaries, using narratives and case studies, and critical incident analysis.

Critical incident analysis

Critical incidents are snapshots or vignettes of an observable activity (a 'moment in time' (Clamp, 1980)), where there is sufficient information to make inferences or predictions about the person who is carrying out the act and the purpose or intention and, importantly, the effects of the act (Flanagan, 1954). Critical incident analysis therefore involves reflecting on either good or bad practice to give insight into that practice. It is not explicitly concerned with identification of ineffective or incompetent practice (Rich and Parker, 1995) as learning can be achieved through the identification and reflection on actions that have had positive outcomes for the care recipient. Benner studied the acquisition of nursing skills and identified critical incidents:

- in which the nurse's intervention made a difference to the care recipients;
- where the outcome went unusually well;
- that led to a breakdown of some kind;
- those that were ordinary and typical;
- that captured the essence of nursing;
- and those that were particularly demanding.

(Benner, 1984)

The use of critical incident analysis as a tool to improve care giving depends on the ability of individuals to reflect upon and question practice and the ability, therefore, of the care giver to recognise either a dissonance between the care given and the required outcome for the care recipient or conversely to recognise why good outcomes were achieved. Throughout this book, case studies will be used as a vehicle for stimulating reflection and critical incidents will be analysed in order to develop learning.

SUMMARY
- The current health policy drivers are focusing on the efficiency and quality of care.
- Professional nursing standards reflect the changing policy focus and the importance of demonstrating different aspects of nursing care such as competence and evidenced-based practice.

- Nursing is both a science and an art. Historically the scientific components have been stressed with a more contemporary theoretical focus on the art of nursing.
- Nursing is a complex activity based on empirics, aesthetic, ethical and personal knowledge.
- Reflective learning is an important way of facilitating transformational learning and helps us to understand nursing principles and practice.

FURTHER READING

Benner, P. (1984) *From novice to expert: excellence and power in clinical nursing practice*. California: Addison-Wesley
This book uses narrative to explore the nature of nursing and the richness of knowledge and skill in nursing practice. Real examples from nursing practice are used throughout, helping the reader to understand the relevance of knowledge and theories within clinical nursing practice.

Daly, J., Speedy, S., Jackson, D. and Darbyshire, P. (eds) (2002) *Contexts of nursing: an introduction*. Oxford: Blackwell
The editors have drawn together a series of chapters that clearly introduce students to concepts relevant to contemporary nursing practice. The book covers a lot of topics, from the history of nursing to research for nursing practice and issues of contemporary relevance, such as the concept of culturally competent care. There is an excellent chapter on the art and science of nursing.

Dingwall, R., Rafferty, A. and Webster, C. (1988) *An introduction to the social history of nursing*. London: Routledge
This book provides a detailed account of the historical development of nursing up until the 1970s and explores the wider social, political and economic developments that impacted on the nature of nursing and its location within the health care system. Different chapters explore different areas of nursing practice development.

Taylor, B. (2000) *Reflective practice: a guide for nurses and midwives*. Buckingham: Open University Press
This book is tailored to the needs of nurses and midwives, and provides an accessible introduction to reflective learning in practice. It offers easy-to-understand definitions of key concepts in reflective practice, as well as a practical guide to the processes of reflection, where types of reflection are applied in different areas of clinical practice.

Chapter 2

An Exploration of the Meaning of Care

The key issues that will be addressed in this chapter are:
- definitions of care and the nature of caring;
- elements of caring and the attributes of the carer;
- caring as a process;
- the relationship between caring and nursing models;
- caring and the therapeutic relationship;
- the measurement and evaluation of care.

By the end of this chapter, you should be able to:
- demonstrate an understanding of the concept of caring;
- discuss the elements that make up a caring person or activity;
- identify the nature of caring within a number of nursing models;
- discuss the importance of care within the therapeutic relationship;
- demonstrate an understanding of the issues and difficulties involved in measuring care.

WHAT IS CARE?

Although in the past 20 years much research into nursing care has been undertaken and caring is considered a core concept in nursing, the concept of caring remains ambiguous. This is also true when considering the nature of caring behaviours. There are a number of definitions of care, but all conclude that care involves more than kind thoughts. Caring is a process and must be demonstrated through actions, which are interpreted by the recipients of care as a particular type of care or non-care (Morrison, 1992).

Activity

Make a list of situations when you have required or may require care. Which individuals would be involved in giving that care?

It can be argued that caring occurs across two settings – the formal economy of care services (including social care and the health service) and the informal economy of care taking place in households and communities (Moullin, 2007). We are mainly concerned here with the formal context of care.

The concept of care

In their examination of the concept of caring, exploring the related literature over 16 years, Brilowski and Wendler (2005, p. 646) noted that descriptions of caring ranged from 'simple stories of exquisitely orchestrated episodes of physical care between a patient and a nurse to rigorous research studies defining and describing the characteristics of professional nurse caring'.

Any core definition of care therefore involves the hands-on approach of physical care giving and something else, which is in the non-physical domain. There is thus a dual nature to caring – attitudes and values towards the care recipient on one hand and activities on the other (McCance *et al.*, 1999).

In order to ensure public safety and meet the organisational goals of health care services when delivering physical care, nurses or care deliverers need to be 'fit for practice' and 'fit for purpose' (United Kingdom Central Council for Nursing, Midwifery and Health Visiting, 1999). This is framed in the ideal of competency. However, physical care giving is not simply about performing a given task, but should be considered in terms of holistic care delivery, with the application of knowledge, skills, values and attitudes within the physical act of doing for the patient.

Activity

Think about an individual that you have cared for, who has required help with washing and dressing.
- What physical care did you perform?
- What non-physical care-giving activities occurred?

It is perhaps the non-physical domain that is the focus of debate in health care settings, as physical care giving or doing for another can be assessed or diagnosed, planned, implemented and evaluated more readily. There are, though, two further aspects to the debate about the nature of caring (Allmark, 1998). Firstly, the cognitive aspect – if one cares about something, one sees it as of value, concern or interest – quite simply one sees some good in it. Secondly, the emotional aspect – if one cares about something, one feels or is disposed to feel an array of emotions in relation to it, like, for example, sorrow or anger at injustice, pity when one fails to thrive.

Activity

Think about how you felt when a marked piece of assessed work was returned to you.
- Did you experience a range of emotions, related to the fact that you cared about the effort that you had put into the work and your progress on the course?
- What emotions did you feel?

Two types of caring needs have been described by Fagerström *et al.* (1998): goal-oriented needs based on scientific knowledge of medicine and then the specifically human needs that require fulfilment for the well-being of people, reducing pain and enhancing well-being. These 'human' needs include:

- belonging to a loving environment;
- education in living in communion with others;
- possibilities for receiving and giving proof of friendship and ten-derness;
- the longing for confirming relationships as having primary im-portance;
- deepest desire of humans for life, love and meaning.

(Fagerström *et al.*, 1998)

Holistic care involves looking beyond physical care needs to human needs, enabling the nurse to have the opportunity to interpret and understand the need for care in its widest context, which is what human beings really need for complete well-being (Eriksson, 1994). Using Maslow's (1962) theory of a hierarchy of needs (see Figure 1), the need to be cared about could be located within safety and security needs as well as belonging needs.

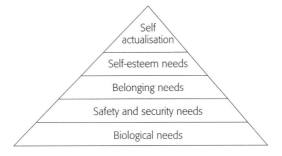

Figure 1 Maslow's (1962) hierarchy of needs

Elements of care

Despite the fact that nurse scholars claim that caring is the foundation of nursing (Stockdale and Warelow, 2000), the concept of care cannot be defined simplistically. Perhaps, instead of trying to rigidly define 'care', we should try to interpret it by examining how to use care in practice and so examine the process of caring. First, in order to provide high-quality care, caring professionals must recognise the different elements of care and have skill and competence in providing care in psychomotor (physical), cognitive (thinking) and affective (emotional) domains (Baillie, 2001). Elements of care could also include those described by Davies and O'Berle (1990) in relation to palliative care but which are relevant to all nurses.

- Valuing, which is about respect for individuals and being non-judgemental.
- Connecting, which is similar to empathising in that it is about listening, understanding, having a caring attitude that says the person is important. Spending time and giving adequate time to care recipients are also aspects of connecting.
- Empowering in terms of enabling self-care and decision-making when possible.
- Finding meaning in terms of what the individual's life is all about, which might involve spiritual assessment.
- Doing for – physical and emotional support, which must involve negotiation not taking over.
- Preserving integrity, not being incapacitated by the emotional effect of caring for another.

Another related element of care is the principle of being person-centred (Talerico, 2003); that is, about knowing the person as an individual and being responsive to their individual characteristics, providing care that is meaningful and respectful of the individual's preferences and values and needs. It also involves fostering consistent and trusting relationships, emphasising freedom of choice including individually defined and reasonable risk taking, promoting comfort, both physical and emotional, and involving the person's family, friends and significant others appropriately.

Activity

What barriers could there be in a ward or community environment to respecting care recipients' personal preferences?
How might trust be compromised?

What attributes does the 'carer' require?

Pryds-Jensen *et al.* (1993) asked 16 nurses to develop a picture of a caring nurse. They included:

- demonstrates knowledge;
- self-confidence;
- knowledge of others;
- timing based on intuition;
- love for humans;
- approach patient with positive attitude;
- committed;
- generous;
- acts calmly to control stressful situation;
- practical skills;
- reflective self-knowledge;
- demonstrates empathy;
- creativity and humour;
- deeply concerned and acts on the basis of ethical values and attitudes;
- honest;
- demonstrates courage.

Rush and Cook (2006) identified the characteristics of care that were valued from a care recipient's point of view to be:

- good communication;
- respect;
- appropriate appearance;
- attention to hygiene;
- detailed knowledge of patients' conditions and treatments.

Brilowski and Wendler (2005) identified five attributes that provide a good framework to consider caring. These were:

- relationship;
- action;
- attitude;
- acceptance;
- variability.

Relationship

When individuals have a relationship they are mutually or reciprocally interested or have a meaningful social relationship (Gove, 1986). Important characteristics of this include trust, intimacy and responsibility

(Moccia, 1988). Trust can be seen in terms of openness, sincerity, love and patience (see the critical incident analysis in Chapter 3). It is important to 'be there' for the person being cared for. It is something about warmth and genuineness, empathetic understanding and unconditional positive regard (Rogers, 1967). In a relationship between a care recipient and care giver, it also involves something about 'knowing the care recipient or "patient"' (Tanner *et al.*, 1993), that is, having an involved rather than a detached understanding of the person's situation and responses, which may be known but may not be able to be described (see the critical incident analysis in Chapter 4). Two broad categories of knowing the patient include knowing their patterns of responses and knowing the patient as a person in quality-of-life terms from the care receiver's perspective. As nurses come to know patients, for example, they are able to express caring as a commitment to protecting the patient's vulnerability while enhancing dignity (see the critical incident analysis in Chapter 7). The professional providing the care needs to be responsible for actions directed towards well-being and therefore knowledge must be current. Professional codes provide the frame for this therapeutic relationship (Russel, 2007) but it goes beyond professionalism and is about being open and honest in terms of congruence between what is being felt and thought and what is being said. It is important to avoid being patronising, or defensive, to not be afraid to give an opinion when appropriate, and be open – this may mean using your own life experiences (Egan, 2002) (see the critical incident analysis in Chapter 4).

Action

Actions involve doing for or being with the care recipient, which originates from the carer's perception of another's need and results in a motivation to act to meet those needs (Fealy, 1995). Important nursing actions include:

- nursing care, with physical care as a primary focus of the interaction;
- touch – a form of non-verbal communication influenced by the nurse's intentionality and the care recipient's perceptions;
- presence – physically and in terms of giving of self, which involved two people occupying the same place;
- competence – an understanding of how human and physical science interacts with the humanity of the care recipient and their family is crucial to good care.

(adapted from Brilowski and Wendler, 2005)

Such actions should be aimed at creating a sense of security and therefore allowing people to be able to pursue everyday activities without having to question what they do (Ousey and Johnson, 2007).

Attitude

Both lay and professional caring behaviours display attributes of commit-ment, knowledge, skills and respect for person (Stockdale and Warelow, 2000). Bjork (1999) argues that it is the intentional elements of practical nursing or care-giving skills that transform practical nursing actions from the acts of handling and helping into tolerable or meaningful experiences for the care recipient. This 'caring about' or presenting a positive attitude towards another could be described as the ontology or 'being' of the nurse. In order for a caring attitude to occur, factors such as trust, rapport, understanding of self and others and commitment have been identified as elements or attributes which need to be present (Brilowski and Wendler, 2005).

Activity

- How can you demonstrate a 'positive' attitude when caring for indivi-duals in a hospital or community environment?
- What barriers might you encounter?

Acceptance

Acceptance is about regarding another person as proper, suitable or normal (Gove, 1986). The most compelling reason that one cares for another is that the other is a fellow human being, worthy of dignity and respect. Nurses attempt to confirm a patient's dignity and support the idea that those in care are intrinsically valuable and precious as human beings (Brilowski and Wendler, 2005). Concern about how a patient views the world is fundamental to nursing and is about helping the indi-vidual on their own terms (Oulton, 1997). This may be about empathetic understanding, where the nurse demonstrates sensitivity for what another person is feeling and conveys this to them (Egan, 2002). This may involve active listening and responding in a way that indicates an understanding of what they are saying.

Central to the caring (or therapeutic) relationship is unconditional accep-tance, where the care giver accepts care recipients as individuals entitled to respect and care without necessarily accepting their values and beha-viours, which may be at odds with one's own value systems (Egan, 2002).

Variability

Variability is the quality of being able to make changes (especially minor or partial changes) or make an attribute or characteristic different (Gove,

1986). This is important because caring is fluid and changing, depending on circumstances, environment and the people involved. Florence Nightingale (1859) stated that nurses must have a conception of the most important thing regarding the patient's situation and because of this it is important that the care giver can respond to such changes in circumstance or priority. In order to achieve this, certain characteristics are required, including:

- respecting the identity and integrity of other human beings;
- being sensitive and non-judgemental;
- knowing when to listen and when to speak;
- having the knowledge and skills to intervene in a way that promotes best quality of life as perceived by the patient.

(Russel, 2007)

Lay perspectives of care and the process of caring

Activity

If you were a patient on a hospital ward, what would be the most important characteristics of the nurses caring for you?

To the general public, nursing and caring are synonymous (Ousey and Johnson, 2007). When health care recipients are asked to describe caring nurses, they include attributes such as being attentive, honest, genuine, involved, good listeners, genuinely concerned about patients' welfare, committed, understanding, respectful of questions, sensitive to patients' needs (Hallsdorsdottir and Hamrin, 1997). In addition, caring is seen as being responsive, respectful, giving a timely response and having confidence in performing procedures (Huycke and All, 2000). Furthermore, in a study in Finland, being cared for entailed experiencing confidence in the competence of the nurses' comfort, guidance, dialogue and closeness. Experiencing pain, discomfort, anxiety, uncertainty and insecurity leads to the need for comfort, trust, security, guidance and above all the need to talk to someone (Fagerström et al., 1998). A longing to be seen, affirmed and understood is important and individuals need to understand their situation.

So, in order to reach people's caring needs, conscious striving and courage are demanded of the nurse in order to look beyond the symptoms of illness and appreciate the individual's perspective of their illness, existence and care needs (Fagerström et al., 1998). Being noticed and well looked after therefore can create a sense of well-being and comfort. The nurse's way of relating is important and should be friendly, pleasant and encouraging, with time spent in dialogue. Guidance and information giving display willingness and create opportunities for contact when the care recipient is experiencing anxiety, insecurity, uncertainty and even depression.

Dissatisfied patients, on the other hand, suffer anxiety and uncertainty, unclear diagnosis, lack of communication and feel they have insufficient guidance. Fagerström *et al.* (1998) identified three deficiencies that might lead to this perception of not being sufficiently cared for:

- Deficiency in the system. Nurses have excessive workload and so do not have time to care.
- Deficiency in the caring culture where the focus of caring today is on identifying symptoms, on illness and its treatment.
- Caring deficiency, where the patient does not feel noticed and understood and will to some extent suffer pain unnecessarily or suffer loneliness.

These issues will be explored in more depth in Chapter 8.

The relationship between care and models of nursing/health care

Both lay and professional caring behaviours display attributes of commitment, knowledge, skills and respect for person (Stockdale and Warelow, 2000). Roach (1984) sees nursing as the professionalisation of human caring, through the affirmation that caring is the human mode of being and through the development of the capacity to care through the acquisition of skills – cognitive, affective, technical and administrative. There is an obligation for the professional nurse to care, as stated in the Nursing and Midwifery Code of Professional Conduct, which requires practitioners to 'make the care of people your first concern, treating them as individuals and respecting their dignity' and also to 'provide a high standard of practice and care at all times' (NMC, 2008, p. 1).

The obligation to care for another human being involves becoming a certain kind of person and not merely doing certain kinds of things. The capacity to perceive and interpret the subjective experiences of others and to imaginatively project the effect of nursing actions in their lives becomes a necessary skill (Carper, 1978), but knowing how to care is not simply a question of skill acquisition but involves a process of unpicking (deconstruction) and rebuilding (reconstruction) in facing the issues presented through the nursing process/process of caring. It is about understanding who we are in the context of defining and understanding nursing practice, having the courage and commitment to change and changing to achieve the desirable practice (Johns, 1995).

The nursing process

Activity

- What are the stages of the nursing process?
- From what you have read so far, identify the ways in which care might fit into these stages.

The nursing process is a plan to get things done (Morse *et al.*, 1990). It is a five-stage problem solving framework, enabling the nurse to plan individualised nursing care for a client. Continually undertaken during a caring episode or over the longer term, the five stages encompass assessment, diagnosis, planning, implementation and evaluation leading on to further assessment or re-assessment. This systematic approach enables nurses to undertake comprehensive, systematic and accurate nursing assessment of the physical, psychological, social and spiritual needs of those in their care and provide a rationale for the care delivered, taking account of the social, cultural, legal, political and economic influences (Hogston and Marjoram, 2007).

Nursing models

Activity

Look at a street, road or railway map. Use it to plan the shortest journey between two points.
What does it tell you about the journey you plan to take or the choices you have when undertaking the journey?

The map provides a visual representation of the area and network of roads, streets and lines. It is not a replica of the system, but provides a schema, so that people can plan journeys and make decisions about which elements of the map are relevant to inform those decisions. If we were to travel between two points on this map, we would only use selected routes and certain points along those lines or roads that would help us to plan our journey. However, seeing these within the context of the whole map helps us to see the broader picture and the way that our particular journey fits with other elements of the system.

The same can be said of nursing models. There are a number of different models, which look at holistic nursing practice from different theoretical perspectives. When using these models, we may select elements of them which are relevant to the individual we are providing care for, so that that care can be individualised and appropriate.

Nursing models therefore go some way towards exploring the delivery of nursing care. Some models focus primarily on the physical aspects of required care, for example the frameworks for assessment created by Roper *et al.* (2000) or 'the activities of living', which involve the nurse caring for the patient by attending to the activities people engage in their daily life.

Roper, Logan and Tierney's activities of daily living (2000)
Maintaining a safe environment.
Communicating.
Breathing.
Eating and drinking.
Eliminating.
Personal cleansing and dressing.
Controlling body temperature.
Mobilising.
Working and playing.
Expressing sexuality.
Sleeping.
Dying.

However, Watson (1985) focuses on the more affective domain of nurse caring in terms of helping people to gain a higher degree of harmony within the mind, body and soul through caring transactions. She describes ten carative factors.

Jean Watson's ten carative factors
Altruistic system of values.
Faith–hope.
Sensitivity to self and others.
Helping–trusting, human care relationship.
Expressing positive and negative feelings.
Creative problem solving caring process.
Transpersonal teaching learning.
Supportive, protective and/or corrective mental, physical, societal and spiritual environment.
Human needs assistance.
Existential–phenomenal–spiritual forces.

(Watson, 1985, p.75)

For Peplau (1952), the focus of nursing was on the therapeutic interpersonal relationship between patient and nurse. Her model is based on humanistic theories and was influenced by prominent psychosocial theorists of the time, such as Freud (1936) and Maslow (1954). Two basic concepts in Peplau's model are anxiety and communication, which she views as interrelated. If communication is seen as threatening in any way, then anxiety results, which is manifested either physically or psychologically. Anxiety is viewed as the energy force of individuals, and the interpersonal relationship has four sequential phases, which help individuals to problem solve and mature emotionally. These phases are:

- orientation, where the nurse makes the care recipient aware of the availability of help;
- identification, where the nurse facilitates the expression of feelings;
- exploitation, where the nurse uses communication skills to help the care recipient view problems realistically, and work to reduce the anxiety so that they may personally grow;
- resolution, where the care recipient becomes independent and disengages from the interpersonal relationship.

The caring role of the nurse in Peplau's model is thus tied up in the interpersonal process and the therapeutic relationship. The humanistic focus of the model requires the nurse to offer unconditional acceptance to individuals, viewing them for what they are. This entails self-awareness and exploration of one's own personal value systems, with personal reflection being an important part of the nurse's development.

Therapeutic relationships

There is little doubt then that the therapeutic relationship is at the heart of caring. Therapeutic relations or the therapeutic use of self are about using self to aid the well-being of an individual. Skilled therapeutic interventions can minimise the psychological morbidity associated with ill health (Russel, 2007). The face-to-face encounter is key in this. When carers do not hear the care recipient's voice, there is a breakdown in our understanding of care and of the kind of relationship upon which care is founded (Peacock and Nolan, 2000). The experience of comfort is created through encouraging words, a comforting touch, sharing the human experience and promoting the physical feeling of comfort through ordinary nursing activities so that a feeling of comfort should be a goal of caring (Gropper, 1992). Therapeutic relations include needing to know self, namely:

- the perception of self feelings and prejudices with the situation;
- the management of the self's feelings and prejudices in order to respond appropriately;

- managing anxiety and sustaining the self (Johns, 1995).

This can be achieved through reflective practice and critical reflection on self.

HOW CAN CARE BE MEASURED?

Activity

Think about your answer to the question:
If you were a patient on a hospital ward, what would be the most important characteristics of the nurses caring for you?
- Could you measure the characteristics you describe?

Measuring care is important on two levels. As stated earlier, nurse caring results in increased health and healing and can result in a sense of solidarity, security, increased self-esteem, increased reality orientation, personal growth and lessening of fear and anxiety for patients (Brilowski and Wendler, 2005). With strong support in the nursing literature for this, then, as a profession, should nurses strive to ensure care is delivered to the highest possible standard by measuring and improving on what is seen?

There are also strong national drivers for the improvement of care delivery, which started with the publication of the White Paper *Working for Patients* (DH, 1989), the NHS Plan (DH, 2000) and *Clinical Governance: Quality in the New NHS* (NHS Executive, 1999), which mandate professionals working in the NHS to improve clinical behaviours in order to improve outcomes for clinical practice. When Labour entered government in 1997, they published a policy called the *New NHS: Modern, Dependable* stating that:

> The new NHS will have quality at its heart. Without it there is unfairness. Every patient who is treated in the NHS wants to know that they can rely on receiving high quality care when they need it. Every part of the NHS, and everyone who works in it, should take responsibility for working to improve quality.
>
> (DH, 1997, pp.3.2).

Clinical governance is 'a framework through which NHS organisations are accountable for improving the quality of their services and safeguarding high standards of care by creating an environment in which excellence in clinical care will flourish' (NHS Executive, 1999). Measuring the 'quality of care' is therefore at the heart of clinical governance and quality-improvement health policy directives.

So how can care be measured?

Care, and therefore quality of care, is a multidimensional concept, which is difficult to measure, as care is always contextualised or understood in context (Warelow, 1996) whether it is a physical, cognitive or affective need. For example, some patients may be embarrassed by the intrusion of care delivery and prefer the nurse to concentrate on the technical task rather than themselves. It is therefore dependent on their encounter with the existing care structure and by their system of norms, expectations and experiences. It can be understood in light of two conditions, the resource structure of the care organisation and the patient's preferences (Wilde Larsson and Larsson, 1999). Therefore of importance are the:

- medical technical competence of the care givers – the ability of the care giver to perform physical care in a safe and competent manner;
- the physical-technical conditions of the care organisation – having the right environment and equipment in order to facilitate care delivery;
- the degree of identity orientation in the attitude and actions of the care givers;
- the socio-cultural atmosphere of the care organisation. See Figure 2.

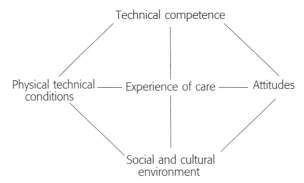

Figure 2 Dimensions of care

The consequences of caring also provide outcome criteria for the assessment of caring in practice (Brilowski and Wendler, 2005). Care can then be measured from perspectives of providers, payers, public and patients (Huycke and All, 2000).

Perspective	Focus
Providers (e.g. health care organisations)	The process and outcomes of care, including having the knowledge to deliver care and achieving the required health outcomes (e.g. meeting waiting-list targets or reducing readmission rates).
Payers (e.g. general public in terms of taxpayers or private insurance)	The affordability and access to care according to need.
Public	Standards and regulation set by the government (using the Health Care Commission's *Standards for Better Health* (Health Care Commission, 2004).
Patients	Subjective view of the quality of care.

Activity

- What might patients want to measure as an indicator of good care?
- What about the health care organisation such as, for example, the hospital or community?

Patients

Patient satisfaction is one factor taken into consideration for judging quality of care (Wilde Larsson and Larsson, 1999). Patients identify the characteristics of quality of care as:

- responsiveness;
- respect;
- timely response;
- confidence in performing procedures.

(Huycke and All, 2000)

Some studies argue that physical care is more important to patients, whereas nurses argue that psychosocial care is more important (Morrison, 1991). Perhaps this reflects Maslow's hierarchy of needs identified earlier, in that this kind of care is only perceived as important when physical needs have been met. Also, could it be argued that patients rely on interpersonal relationships to evaluate health care as they lack the technical knowledge to make judgements about quality of care itself? Put another way, the care receiver is not able to judge the quality of a physical intervention such as heart surgery, and so relies on the interpersonal care or feelings of security or being 'cared for' as a measure of quality.

Donabedian (1966) describes a model of quality assurance for the evaluation of health care and describes three approaches to specifying and measuring quality: structure, process and outcome. He noted that all three are equally important in measuring the quality of care provided by a health care organisation and that they are complementary and should be used collectively to monitor quality of care. 'Structure' refers to human and physical resources and can include staff and policy. 'Process' refers to the methods of working, so may include the procedures for allocating resources or implementing clinical guidelines. 'Outcomes' refer to the effect of both the structure and the process, the result of a number of individual 'outputs'. The outcome relating to a clinical guideline being introduced would be improved patient care with improved clinical outcomes. The assumption inherent in the model is that if structure and process are right, then the desired outcomes will result.

Nurses measuring caring

The evaluation of nursing care must be an ongoing process and can be achieved through activities such as:

- nursing handover – the chance to discuss care and its effectiveness;
- reflection – the belief that self can be developed to be used more effectively within a person's practice by reflecting on and in action (Johns, 1995);
- patient satisfaction;
- reviewing the nursing plan – have goals been achieved?

(Hogston and Marjoram, 2007)

Carper's (1978) four patterns of knowing can also provide pathways through which the fullness of the nursing situation can be known (Boykin and Schoenhofer, 1991).

Empirical knowing

Empirical elements include those that are factual, objectively describable and generalisable. They enable the systematic review of the outcomes of care but cannot, however, stand alone due to the context of specific clinical situations – unforeseen human responses.

Case study

Unforeseen human responses

A tissue viability team may introduce a new type of wound dressing based on evidence from research of its efficacy. The team may audit the use of this dressing against standards such as length of healing time and cost. Despite this, however, the team may not be able to account for the individual care recipient who will not accept the new approach as he/she has always used the old dressing type historically and can't understand why the change is necessary, as it has 'always worked for me'. As a result, and despite being given the objective facts about the new dressing type, this individual peels it back and checks the wound daily to monitor the situation, thereby introducing infection and negating the occlusive effect of the dressing, thus impeding healing.

Aesthetics

Aesthetics involves the process of perceiving or grasping the nature of a clinical situation, interpreting this information in order to understand its meaning for all involved and envisioning desired outcomes in order to respond with appropriate and skilled action (Johns, 1995). This can be achieved through reflective practice.

In the case study above the aesthetic approach may result in the tissue viability team revisiting the recommendation for dressing change. The team may spend more time with the individual, giving information and reassurance and actually making judgements as to whether, in this case, it would be more appropriate to resort to the old dressing type.

Empathy

Empathy is a key skill here for this interpretation of the clinical situation. Empathy is the ability to enter the perceptual world of another person and see the world as they see it, but also that there is an element of conveying this understanding to the person (Burnard, 1990). When the nurse reflects on the person, has that connectivity been established? This is about nurses striving to give what Noddings (1984) describes as motivational shift. That is, they are not simply motivated by the ethical principles but by the ideal of caring itself, based on understanding the patient's reality as a possibility for oneself.

Activity

In our brief case study above this might mean the nurse trying to under-stand why the individual feels as she does. For example, think about issues of choice and control in this case study.

Ethics

Caring as an ethical foundation for nursing is a moral stance; it is about protection, enhancement and preservation of human dignity (Watson, 1985). There are four ethical principles:

- autonomy – the right of a person to make their own decisions and direct their life;
- beneficence – the responsibility of doing good and so providing benefit or beneficial treatment/care to the person;
- non-maleficence – the responsibility of avoiding harm to the person;
- justice – the responsibility to be equitable and fair in the way we treat others.

It is also important when determining appropriate ethical action that the practitioner always pays attention to conflicts of values within themselves and between themselves and others.

Activity

In our case study it is important to try to understand whether the clinical decision to make a wound dressing change in this case is actually resulting in harm to the individual. An individual may be unable to grasp the rationale for the changes imposed, responds in a way that may actually worsen the clinical problem presenting, and will become anxious and lose all trust in the nursing team trying to help her.

However, as a word of warning, it is important to recognise that, in considering caring as purely moral, the act becomes an obligation and so there is an immediate responsibility to care for the patient according to his or her needs regardless of the nurse's abilities or the patient's characteristics or receptivity (Stockdale and Warelow, 2000). For exam-ple, a situation where a patient refuses care when this refusal may actually result in harm or even death (e.g. refusing blood transfusion). Also writers have described 'habitualisation' – that is, routine and coping-dominated practice, when a condition is very familiar to the nurse so that they lose compassion and do not listen to patients fully (Heath, 1998).

So, as our case study illustrates, if our thinking is underpinned entirely by the scientific/technological (empirical) domain of knowing, everything, including care, can be measured objectively. Calculation and results become the frame through which the world is measured. We speak of quality of health care provision but mean only what can be calculated, weighed and assessed. Caring interventions must be written down as plans with quantifiable outcomes and demonstrate value for money. What is required, though, is a philosophy of caring within which the scientific/technological can take its proper place supplementary to more fundamental forms of caring (Peacock and Nolan, 2000, p. 1069) and Carper's ways of knowing offers a clear frame for this through the reflective practice ideal.

SUMMARY
- Caring is multifaceted and is a complex concept to define.
- Caring is integral to nursing and the therapeutic relationship.
- Caring can be physical, emotional and psychological.
- Measurement of care depends on the context and focus of the purpose.
- It is easier to measure care that can be objectively viewed, although elements of the caring relationship may be as important or more important.

FURTHER READING

Hogston, R. and Marjoram, B.A. (2007) *Foundations of nursing practice: leading the way*. Hampshire: Palgrave MacMillan
This book lays down a broad base of knowledge, covering the physical and psychological sides of nursing care. It is clearly written, supported by both simple illustrations and activities, and each chapter has summaries, tests and generic case studies as well as useful references and further reading sections.

Egan, G. (2006) *The skilled helper: a problem-management and opportunity-development approach to helping*. London: Thomson Learning
This book emphasises the collaborative nature of the therapist–client relationship and uses a practical, three-stage helping model that drives client problem-managing and opportunity-developing action. It focuses on evidence-based practice, research and philosophical perspectives around how helpers know what they know and is highly applicable to the nursing context.

Brophy, S., Snooks, H. and Griffiths, L. (2008) *Small-scale evaluation in health: a practical guide*. London: Sage

This book sets out the basics of designing, conducting and analysing an evaluation study in health care. A practical approach is taken and the authors assume no previous knowledge or experience of evaluation in the reader. All the basics are covered, including: how to plan an evaluation; research governance and ethics; understanding data; interpreting findings; and writing a report. There are cases included throughout to demonstrate evaluation in action and self-learning courses give the reader an opportunity to develop their skills further in the methods and analysis involved in evaluating health care.

Chapter 3

Mental Health, Interpersonal Relationships and Psychosocial Care

The key issues that will be addressed in this chapter are:

- interpersonal skills and communication;
- issues of confidentiality;
- engagement and disengagement between carer and care recipient;
- the concept of stigma and stigma management;
- the context of mental health care provision.

By the end of the chapter you will be able to:

- identify critical incidents from a case study;
- use Gibbs' reflective cycle to examine a critical incident;
- analyse the case study using frameworks of knowledge to identify relevant issues in the care of people with mental health problems;
- use Peplau's model of nursing to consider the caring process;
- consider issues of the therapeutic relationship in the process of care;
- consider how the care provided in this case study could be evaluated.

INTRODUCTION

The case study in this chapter explores the experience of a man who became depressed after a series of life events led him to turn to work for solace and then to alcohol. It reflects the work that a nurse might undertake when working with people who have mental health problems. It is estimated that, in any one year, one in four British adults will experience at least one diagnosable mental health problem, with mixed anxiety and depression being the most commonly diagnosed disorder. Between 8 and 12 per cent of the adult British population will be diagnosed with depression in any one year (Office for National Statistics Psychiatric Morbidity Report, 2001). Of the people diagnosed with mental health problems, about half are no longer affected after 18 months, but people from poorer backgrounds, the long-term sick and the unemployed are more likely to be affected for longer periods of time than other members of the population (Office for National Statistics, 2003).

In mental health nursing there has been a recognition of the need for access to earlier intervention and greater access to the talking therapies that support self care in order to prevent individuals spiralling into the reality of long-term mental health issues, dependency on drugs (prescribed or illegal) or alcohol or contemplation of suicide.

In order to support mental health and psychosocial care needs, the nurse caring for the individual in this case study will work holistically across a range of care settings, but importantly in the care recipient's home in order to build on his strengths to facilitate recovery and optimise health and well-being (DH, 2007b). The majority of people with symptoms of depression are cared for within a community setting (Thomas *et al.*, 1996).

Summary of the role of the community mental health team
- Giving advice on management of mental health problems (especially to the PHCT and providing triage function for referral).

Providing treatment and care for those:
- with time-limited disorders who will benefit from specialist interventions;
- providing treatment and care for those with more complex and enduring mental health needs.

(DH, 2002b)

The ultimate goal of the intervention is to promote self-care through advice, information or treatment for illness or disturbances in mental health and well-being. The case study demonstrates the successful organisation of care, recognition of Peter's specific need for 'care' in the cognitive and emotional domains and the comfort and emotional strength for recovery provided by a skilled nurse who successfully 'cared' for him. Peter's depression can be termed reactive depression, where his symptoms emerged as a reaction to specific events in his life (Bonham, 2004). The nurse enabled recognition and validation of symptoms and therefore helped Peter to address some of the mental health issues he was experiencing. A community psychiatric nurse (CPN) who is a member of the community mental health team (CMHT) is providing the care in this case.

THE MENTAL HEALTH, INTERPERSONAL RELATIONSHIPS AND PSYCHOSOCIAL CARE CASE STUDY

(Peter's story)

I don't know how I felt when the doctor diagnosed me with depression.

In some ways, it was a relief because, although I didn't want to admit it I hadn't been coping very well for a few weeks. At least having the label gave some reason for my symptoms, and gave me some hope that I would get better.

It started when Florence, my long-term partner, left me for another man. I didn't want people to feel sorry for me or think I was weak, so I threw myself into my work as a sales representative for a pharmaceutical company, which was not difficult as there was always plenty to do. I volunteered for extra responsibilities, and soon ended up working longer and longer hours, in order to keep up with everything. I started having a couple of glasses of whisky at night, to relax me before going to bed, but still found myself waking in the early hours of the morning. Friends now tell me how worried they were, as I had lost over a stone in weight because I was not eating properly, and was pale and tired and was too frequently under the influence of alcohol. As I became more and more tired, I struggled to motivate myself to get up in the morning, and one day when I was driving home, I had a panic attack, which really frightened me.

A close friend encouraged me to go and see my GP, who diagnosed me with depression. She prescribed some anti-depressants, which she said would help me to manage the symptoms in the short-term, although I wasn't too keen on taking them. She also referred me to a community psychiatric nurse for some counselling.

I was very anxious on the first day that I met the CPN. I was used to being in control of my life, and now I was feeling very vulnerable, unable to make decisions and not sure what I was doing. While there is a lot about this period of my life that I don't remember, I do remember the first meeting with the CPN, George. He came to my house and we sat in the kitchen, while I made coffee. I don't know what I was expecting, but George sat and chatted with me for a while. It was a bit like talking to a mate, as we chatted about football and music. I don't know why I felt so comfortable with George, but I felt that I could trust him.

After we had chatted for a while, George said that he was required to make notes about his visit, but assured me of confidentiality and that anyone who had access to these notes would not be able to trace them to me. This was very important to me as, with my job, I sometimes had to visit the local hospitals and surgeries and did not want to feel compromised in my role. I also felt able to ask him about the anti-depressants that the doctor had prescribed and he reassured me about their use and answered questions about the side-effects that I might experience. As a result of this discussion, I decided that I would take them.

George arranged to see me on a weekly basis. One week, he asked me to draw a biographical timeline, identifying important points in my life. I found this really hard, and had a very emotional week. At the end of the next visit, I told George that I didn't seem to have done very much over the preceding week. He immediately disagreed with me, and said that he thought that I had worked very hard emotionally, and he recognised the impact that this had had on me. I felt validated by this, and felt that George really understood what I was experiencing.

Although I can't really remember the details of all the counselling sessions that I had with George, I did realise how he helped me to work through some of the issues that had contributed to my depression. We spent a long time talking about my father, and he helped me to realise how I had continually striven to live up to my father's expectations, and how I had placed unrealistic demands on myself, as I constantly strove for perfection, thinking that what I was doing was not quite good enough. We also talked about my relationship with Florence (my ex-girlfriend), and he helped me to see how I had also chased an idealistic dream of perfection. I realised that I couldn't have a successful relationship with someone else while I was not being true to myself.

After some weeks, George said that he thought that it was time to cease the counselling sessions. I had been negotiating my phased return to work, and George suggested that I was ready to try and cope without the counselling. However, he said that I could contact him at any time if I felt that I wanted to discuss anything with him, or if I wanted to recommence the counselling. This was very important to me, as I was very anxious about how I was going to cope, but knowing that I could contact George made me feel safer.

Critical incident analysis exercise

Using critical incident analysis, as described at the end of Chapter 1, can you list all the elements from this case study that could be described as a critical incident? Include examples of practice that were either good or bad as well as incidents that can give insight into practice, focusing specifically on why it was successful or could have been improved in some way. Give at least three positive examples and an example where the nurse could have improved the outcome for the service user. You may wish to refer to the work of Benner detailed in Chapter 1, but particularly think about incidents:

- in which the nurse's intervention made a difference to the care recipient;

- that were ordinary and typical;
- that captured the essence of nursing.

(Benner, 1984)

Commentary on the case study

The following is a list of the possible critical incidents that could be used for reflection on this case study. These have been mapped to the attributes and characteristics that service users valued in nurses as presented by Rush and Cook (2006) and Pryds-Jensen *et al.*'s (1993) attributes of a 'caring nurse'.

Possible critical incident	Commentary	Rush and Cook (2006) and Pryds-Jensen *et al.* (1993) attributes and characteristics
The first meeting with George, the CPN.	This was important, as rapport and trust were established.	Communication. Approach the patient with a positive attitude. Competence.
The fact that the meeting was at Peter's house, sitting in the kitchen while Peter made coffee.	This was normalising and gave Peter some control and comfort as it was in his social environment.	Competence. Respect. Communication. Approach the patient with a positive attitude. Committed. Honest. Generous. Demonstrate courage. Acts calmly to control stressful situations.
Information-giving about the anti-depressants.	This demonstrated knowledge, but was also important in terms of compliance.	Detailed knowledge of the patient's condition and treatments. Competence. Honest.
Validation of the care recipient's feelings after the completion of the timeline.	George demonstrated empathy and understanding here, but also empowered Peter and boosted his self-esteem. There was validation here of the emotional work that Peter had undertaken.	Demonstrate empathy. Knowledge of others. Approach patient with a positive attitude. Competence. Communication.
Counselling sessions exploring the care recipient's relationship with his father and his ex-girlfriend.	George helped Peter to find solutions to problems, which was empowering and enabled growth.	Self-confidence. Honest. Competence. Knowledge. Communication.
The decision to terminate the sessions.	This was very important to Peter as the anxiety about how he was going to cope could have become debilitating. Knowing that he could contact George made him feel safer during the time when he was re-establishing his emotional independence. The timing of disengagement is important, so that the recipient can be empowered to be self-supporting.	Timing based on intuition. Demonstrate courage. Self-confidence. Competence. Knowledge of others. Demonstrates empathy. Approach patient with positive attitude. Committed.

There are other possible critical incidents:

- Peter felt it was a bit like talking to a mate chatting about football and music, which helped him to feel comfortable with George so that he could trust him.
- Peter realised how George helped him to work through some of the issues that had contributed to his depression.
- Peter was relieved at being given the diagnosis of depression. Having the label gave some rationale for his symptoms, and gave him hope that he would get better.

Exercise using Gibbs' Reflective Cycle

Use Gibbs' reflective learning cycle (see Chapter 1) to reflect on one of the critical incidents that you have identified. Work through the stages of the cycle, ensuring you include the actions that you would take to improve user outcomes in the future. This may relate to improving the outcomes for this particular care recipient, or replicating positive actions in this scenario for other care recipients.

Physical, cognitive and emotive domains or aspects

Activity

Can you think of examples of care given within this case study that fit within the:
- Physical domain?
- Cognitive domain?
- Emotive domain?

Physical domain

At first glance, it seems that there are no physical components of care giving within this case study. However, George uses his knowledge about medication and the physical impact of medication so that Peter can make an informed decision about concordance with the medication regime. This is important, not only in terms of the reassurance that is provided to Peter so that he feels comfortable to comply with the regime (Nettleton, 2006), but also demonstrates sound knowledge of the medicine's actions, risks and benefits according to the criteria set out in the NMC clusters (ESC 36:ii). In doing this, George uses evidence about the efficacy of medications to provide Peter with relevant information (Gomm and Davies, 2000). There are also elements of physical care giving within the communication process, in terms of eye contact, physical touch and body language (Heron, 2001; Burnard, 1994; Bonham, 2004) (**KSF Core dimension 1; ESC 6.i; 6.ii**).

Cognitive domain

Care in the cognitive domain can be seen in the shared search for meaning about how Peter was feeling and George's validation of his emotions. Through this, George demonstrates a commitment to Peter and values him as a person. The therapeutic relationship that George and Peter engage in then helps Peter to see the value of his emotions and his own self-worth (see below).

Emotive domain

George also values the emotional work that Peter engages with and, rather than dismissing this, helps Peter to recognise this emotion. The use of the timeline is a tool that George uses to enable Peter to identify emotional aspects of his life, and ways to cope with these. Thus George helps Peter to 'own' his emotions, and facilitates self-care so that Peter can become more emotionally independent

Analysing the caring process using frameworks of knowledge

Working through a critical incident or using Gibbs' reflective cycle enables us to recognise how important it is to understand the knowledge that underpins an activity so that we can understand the way in which that knowledge is organised and applied in practice. In order to do this the physical, cognitive and emotive domains of nursing and Carper's four fundamental patterns of knowing that underpin contemporary nursing practice will be explored.

One of the key skills that George uses in his interactions with the service user is his communication skills. Good communication is at the heart of nursing care, and many theorists and researchers stress the importance of interpersonal relationships in the therapeutic relationship with care recipients (Peplau, 1952; Burnard, 1999; Meredith *et al.*, 2001).

Within nursing, interpersonal communication is used as a planned activity to help individuals and families to prevent or cope with illness, and sometimes to help people to find meaning within the experience (Lindberg *et al.*, 1990) and, as such, involves guiding, planning and purposefully directing the interaction (**ESC 1.v; 2.iii**). This is particularly relevant here, as George uses his communication and interpersonal skills to help Peter to engage with the problems that contributed to his depression, and to find solutions for himself within his own personal framework. Although Peter says that it is 'a bit like talking to a mate', there is a difference between the communication between friends and the communication in a caring encounter. The communication in friendships and in the practitioner/ client encounter share commonalities in that they both involve social engagement, warmth and mutual enjoyment, but it is the fact that the communication in nursing is a purposeful activity with a planned outcome that distinguishes it. Thus communication is used as a therapeutic intervention in the nurse's helping relationship with the client involving talking, advising and counselling (Burnard, 1994).

Counselling skills are an essential component of mental health nursing work although, as Stickley (2002) points out, there is a difference between being a counsellor and using counselling skills. Nurses use counselling skills as part of a repertoire of skills, while professional counsellors have undertaken a distinct programme of counselling training and their work involves a unitary focus on listening, reflecting feelings and meanings and, at times, offering interpretations to the client (Stickley, 2002). Nevertheless, counselling skills are an important element in the mental health nurse's armoury of skills and provision of care (Burnard, 1999) (**ESC 5**).

> Counselling is the process of sitting and talking to a client, patient or colleague with the intention of helping them to arrive at decisions about how to act.
>
> (Burnard, 1994, p. 62)

Burnard goes on to say that this involves both listening skills and skilled interventions.

Activity

From this case study, can you identify episodes where George uses listening skills and skilled interventions?

Carper's *Fundamental Patterns of Knowing in Nursing*

Communication can be both a science and an art, in that it has an empirical element as well as an aesthetic quality. Additionally, there are ethical dimensions of communication demonstrated within this case study, and George uses his personal knowledge to develop trust, rapport and problem-solving strategies.

Empirics

Communication within a professional–client relationship is not an innate activity, but it is a skill, which can be learned. The empirical component of communication is concerned with the concepts of good communication and the development of skills. Shannon and Weaver (1949) have proposed a model of communication that has been used as a basis for explaining communication in a diverse range of fields (Wood, 2004). This involves a process where a message is sent via a signal from a source and is received at a destination.

This seems quite straightforward but, within this linear pattern of communication, there are a number of potential barriers between the message being sent and received, meaning the message can be distorted.

Activity

Get a group of people together and sit in a circle. Using the game of 'Chinese whispers', get one person to whisper a message to the person on their left, who will then pass on the message to the person on their left, and so on. Continue this process until the message arrives at the last person in the circle, who will say the message out loud.
- Has the message been distorted in any way as it travelled around the circle?
- What are the barriers that might have affected the transition of the message?
- Make a list of the potential barriers in the transmission of the message between nurse and care recipient.

While Shannon's model is useful in demonstrating the process of the transmission of a simple message between two people, it is problematic for the explanation of the complexity of communication within a health care encounter. It fails to take account of the two-way process of communication. In face-to-face contact in the interpersonal relationship, a caring health care professional will not only transmit a message, but will also assess the impact of that message on the receiver, who will give messages back to the sender. The senders and receivers of messages will use more than one strategy and signal to transmit a message. Therefore, verbal communication is not just about words, but includes a whole range of other sounds, gestures, facial expressions and body language.

> **Activity**
>
> **Role play**
>
> Get into a group of three people.
> The first person should try to explain a new skill to a second person.
> The role of the third person is to observe the interaction and make a note of all the different communication strategies that the other two people use.

Burnard (1994) summarises the aspects of communication as linguistic aspects (words, phrases, metaphors), paralinguistic aspects (timing, accent, 'ums and ers', fluency), and non-verbal aspects (eye contact, body language, touch, gesture, etc).

There is also empirical evidence of the benefits of allowing people to talk, so that the nurse is able to hear the care recipient's narrative, which contextualises their suffering within the context of their lives. This helps the nurse to understand the situation from the care recipient's perspective as well as identifying resources that they may have to address the problems. Therefore, rather than being an unstructured activity, story-telling is a purposeful and planned process, based on sound empirical evidence (Fredrikkson and Lindstrom, 2002).

Aesthetics

The art of communication within the caring relationship can be seen in the personal style of the communication and the intuitive understanding of the care recipient. George demonstrates this through his initial contact with Peter, where he demonstrates an empathetic understanding of Peter's anxiety and creatively uses communication to develop a rapport and put Peter at ease. While the conversation about football and music can be seen as general chit-chat, this is in fact a skilled encounter, where George engages with topics of conversation that are familiar to Peter to develop this rapport. There is a difference between thoughtful and thoughtless communication, based on the notion of intention (Heron, 2001). Far from being general chat, this communication demonstrates planning and intention in the development of the interpersonal relationship (**ESC 5.iii**).

Three phases of growth can be identified in the interpersonal communication of the nurse/client relationship.

1. **Opening (initial)** – this is the phase where the two participants adapt to each other and develop trust in each other. Within this case study, we can see that both Peter and George use communication to establish contact and adapt to each other. Peter takes on the role of host, while George uses his skills to establish rapport through chatting about football and music. This is important, as it involves discussion of familiar topics for Peter and reduces some of his anxieties about the counselling sessions.

2. **Working (developmental)** – this phase of the therapeutic encounter involves strategies to help the care recipient to grow, to identify ways of problem-solving and decision-making. We can see in this case that George uses counselling skills and strategies to help Peter to explore his feelings and the issues that have contributed to his current depression. An example of this is the biographical timeline that George asks Peter to complete.

3. **Closing (terminating)** – this phase involves not only the disengagement of the practitioner, but the redirection of trust, so that the client is no longer dependent on the practitioner. Within this case study, George uses his skill to initiate disengagement but, sensing the anxiety that Peter might have in redirecting his trust, shows his empathy and caring by providing the life-line that Peter can contact him if he has any problems. This is empowering, as it enables Peter to take control over the decision-making process.

Ethical knowledge

George demonstrates an ethical dimension of nursing knowledge, through his respect for Peter's confidentiality, self-respect and dignity. Although he needs to keep records of the meetings for accountability, he remains sensitive to Peter's feelings and operates within the NMC's Code (2008). **(Essence of Care Benchmark – Record Keeping)**.

As a registered nurse, midwife or health visitor, you are personally accountable for your practice.

This requires you to:

i. Respect people's confidentiality:
   • You must respect people's right to confidentiality;
   • You must ensure people are informed about how and why information is shared by those who will be providing their care.

ii. Work effectively as part of a team

iii. Manage risk

The Code: Standards of Conduct, Performance and Ethics for Nurses and Midwives (NMC, 2008)

Personal knowledge

Burnard (1992) argued that first impressions are important in social situations, and this is particularly significant when examining the process of interpersonal relationships in the caring encounter. Awareness of self is therefore important, as within any interpersonal encounter the presentation of self will influence the relationship and rapport.

Activity

Think about a situation when you met someone for the first time.
- What did you like or dislike about that person when you met them?
- Reflect on how this might have affected the development of the relationship.

Activity

Your boyfriend/girlfriend has just told you that they want to split after you have been seeing each other for several months. You had no idea that there were problems with the relationship and you are devastated. You have an important piece of coursework to complete, but are having problems concentrating. You go to see your tutor to discuss this with them.
- Reflect on this scenario.

The tutor says that they are very busy and can only spare a couple of minutes. They invite you to sit in the chair on the other side of their desk and ask what the problem is. As you start to explain the situation, they are distracted by an incoming email on their computer. Although they do not open the email, they are constantly flicking their eyes onto the computer screen.
- How would you feel in this situation?

What would make you feel more comfortable disclosing your emotions to them?

An open and empathic approach encourages effective listening and trust and honesty in the practitioner/client relationship (Burnard, 1994). Egan (2002) used the acronym SOLER to help practitioners to develop skills of awareness of their presentation of self when communicating with others. SOLER refers to:

Sitting with an
Open posture
Leaning forward, using appropriate
Eye contact and being
Relaxed.

Although we do not have details of George's presentation of self within this case study, it is clear that Peter's first impressions of him are favourable as he identifies that he felt comfortable with him and that he could trust him. This is important in the development of the relationship and George's subsequent ability to engage with Peter in a therapeutic way (**ESC 5.v**).

Therapeutic use of self

The concept of self is important within health care encounters. People who engage with health services may have a damaged concept of self, either because of physiological or psychological changes. Stigma is an important concept for understanding this damaged concept of self for people who have been diagnosed with a mental health problem.

> Stigma may be defined as a negative social reaction. It also reflects
> social devaluation and negative labelling of individuals.
> (Moon and Gillespie, 1995, p. 88)

The notion of labelling is relevant here, as it is the diagnostic label that marks the person out as different, and leads to the negative social reaction. There is much evidence that lay people still have a poor understanding of mental illnesses and those with diagnosed mental illnesses are stigmatised by society (Clarke, 2001). The negative devaluing of people with stigmatised conditions therefore has an impact, as the stigma may lead to a mismatch between actual social identity and perceived social identity, with damaging effects on their self-esteem.

The term 'therapeutic use of self' is a term that is influenced by nursing theorists from the humanistic perspective (e.g. Peplau – see below) and involves the use of self in the therapeutic alliance to help clients to re-engage with their authentic self, and to rediscover their self-esteem and self-regard (Freshwater, 2002). Thus, within the therapeutic encounter, nurses need to be self-aware and genuine, so that they can use social interaction and reflective processes to enable the care recipient to rediscover their genuine self.

> When a nurse uses self therapeutically she consciously makes use of
> her personality and knowledge in order to effect a change in the ill
> person. This change is seen as therapeutic when it alleviates the
> individual's stress.
> (Travelbee, 1971, p. 19)

Within the case study, we can see how George uses his personality and knowledge to develop a trusting relationship with Peter, and to enable Peter to rediscover his own genuine self and coping mechanisms.

Emotional labour

Another aspect of self-awareness and personal knowledge in the caring relationship is the concept of emotional labour. Hochschild (1983) first developed the concept in relation to flight attendants, where she refers to emotional labour as: 'the management of feeling to create a publicly observable facial and bodily display' (p. 7).

Emotional labour involves the display of certain emotions in order to appear genuine and authentic within the helping role. This concept has been developed in relation to nursing practice by a number of authors (Smith, 1992; James, 1989; Henderson, 2001) focusing on the relationship between emotional attachment/detachment and subjectivity/objectivity in relation to nursing care. According to Henderson (2001), this seems to be tied to knowledge of self and self-management and varies between different clients/patients and circumstances. Within this case study, we can see that George demonstrates an emotional attachment to Peter through his empathic understanding and validation of Peter's feelings and discussion of relationships, and yet maintains a professional distance and objectivity so that he can help Peter to identify problems and make decisions. Similarly, George demonstrates an objective detachment in the decision to disengage from the relationship, when he uses his professional judgement to suggest that Peter no longer needs to see him while, at the same time, demonstrating an emotional attachment and understanding of Peter's anxieties about this disengagement (**Essence of Care Benchmark – Principles of Self Care; ESC 2.v**).

Thus interpersonal communication is fundamental to the caring relationship, and involves physical, cognitive and emotive domains, as well as the four fundamental patterns of knowing as identified by Carper (1978):

> Locked in each person is a wealth of unique experiences, strengths, feelings and values. Effective communication is the master key that unlocks such human resources, enabling a nurse to understand, to care, and to help another person.
>
> (Lindberg *et al.*, 1990, p. 251)

Peplau's model of nursing

Peplau is seen as a key theorist in mental health nursing. For Peplau, nursing is a therapeutic healing art and the interpersonal relationship is central to this. Her model is based on humanistic theories and was influenced by prominent psychosocial theorists of the time, such as Freud and Maslow. Two basic concepts in Peplau's model are anxiety and communication, which she views as interrelated. If communication is seen as threatening in any way, then anxiety results, which is manifested either physically or psychologically.

Anxiety is viewed as the energy force of individuals, and the interpersonal relationship has four sequential phases, which help individuals to problem-solve and mature emotionally. This therapeutic relationship involves the mutual pursuit of the goal, within which the nurse will assume different roles as the relationship develops. This interpersonal relationship is seen as a dynamic learning experience for both nurse and client, where the nurse finds out how the client understands and experiences the felt need, and acts as a resource person, teacher or counsellor to help the client to understand their experiences and to foster social and personal growth. Peplau's sequential stages of the interpersonal relationship are:

- orientation;
- identification;
- exploitation;
- resolution.

Orientation phase

There are two characteristics of the orientation phase. A health need has been identified and professional assistance is thought to be helpful. This help might be immediately needed (as in the case of someone presenting as an emergency) or it might be something that is more planned. Within this case study, we can see how Peter expressed his felt need to a friend following his panic attack and how the friend helped him to see that he needed some professional help. This help was something that was planned, as he first went to see his GP and then arrangements were made for him to see the CPN. Within the orientation phase, the nurse makes the client aware of the availability of help.

Identification phase

Within the identification phase, the nurse facilitates the expression of feelings. The client may respond in one of three ways: independent person, apart from the nurse; independent person in relationship with the nurse; person dependent on the nurse (Ryan Belcher and Brittain Fish, 1990).

Activity

Which response do you think Peter demonstrated in this case study?

In facilitating the expressions of feelings, it is important that the nurse values the person and does not invalidate or reject the person. Thus, an important part of the caring relationship is non-judgementalism. This reflects a humanistic perspective of caring, often associated with the work of Carl Rogers (1967). He argued that an accepting, empathic and non-judgemental approach would help many people to use their own inherent drive towards positive resolution of a problem. Thus the role of the nurse is to facilitate self-help, rather than to direct the person and determine the nature of that help.

Exploitation phase

This is the major phase of Peplau's model of caring, where the nurse, through the use of communication, helps the client to realistically understand their problem, with the goal of reducing their anxiety. Within this case study, we can see how George facilitates Peter's realistic understanding of his problems and anxieties through the use of the timeline and the exploration of his relationships (particularly with his father and his ex-girlfriend). Through this understanding, Peter then develops strategies and decision-making to reduce his anxieties.

Resolution phase

This phase is where the client disengages from the nurse, redirecting their trust and becoming more independent. Again, we can see this as Peter independently negotiates his phased return to work before George suggests that they should cease the counselling sessions.

For Peplau, nursing care is therefore fundamentally concerned with the interpersonal relationship. Nurse and client may come from very different backgrounds and understandings, and the therapeutic relationship involves the pursuit of a mutual goal. As the relationship develops, there is greater shared understanding of roles and therefore more collaborative working. Throughout the phases of the therapeutic relationship, the nurse may adopt a number of different roles, including:

- teacher;
- resource;
- counsellor;
- leader;
- technical expert;
- surrogate.

Activity

Identify episodes where George adopts these different roles in the case study.

THE EVALUATION OF CARE

The discussion so far has identified a number of theoretical frameworks for identifying and analysing elements of the caring process in this case study, particularly focusing on the importance of communication and the interpersonal process in the provision of care. But how can the care be evaluated? One way to consider the success of this care episode is to use Huycke and All's (2000) evaluative framework, which considers outcomes of care from the perspective of providers, payers, public and patients. This is not dissimilar to the outcomes framework identified within the Department of Health *Positive Practice Guide* (2007b), which identifies the benefits of psychological therapies and advocates improved access to them.

Health and well-being outcomes framework	
Patient experience	Inclusion (including employment)
Choice and access	Health and well-being

(Department of Health, 2007b)

Providers

From the provider's perspective, the care in this scenario can be evaluated positively, in that the appropriate level of care is given within the community, fitting in with contemporary policy imperatives of self-help, facilitation and health promotion. From George's personal viewpoint as the provider of nursing care, there is also a positive outcome, as he uses his skills effectively to provide evidence-based care, leading to resolution of Peter's problems and the achievement of the goal of independence.

Payers

Value for money and effective use of resources are important measures of the outcomes of care for payers. Although there have been relatively few studies into the economic benefits of community care in mental health, in their study in 1983 Mangen *et al.* demonstrated that it was cheaper for CPNs to provide aftercare than psychiatrists. In addition, Peter had access to appropriate and timely care, thus reducing the likelihood of a progressive worsening of symptoms and the need for more intensive treatment. George's interventions and focus on problem-solving and self-help may also have reduced the likelihood of repeat episodes and need for longer-term support.

Public

The benefits of community care are measured not only in terms of economic efficiencies for payers, but also in terms of the benefits for the wider community. Gournay and Brooking (1995) identified net benefits to the community through the use of CPNs in working with people with less serious mental health problems. This economic benefit was most noticeable in the reduction in absenteeism from work, although less tangible in other outcome measures.

Patients

Within this case study, we can see that there may be subjective elements of care that Peter would evaluate positively. As discussed throughout this chapter, the nature of the interpersonal process is important and, in particular, the validation of Peter's feelings and emotions, thus contributing to his self-esteem and helping him to identify solutions to his problems. In addition, the non-judgementalism of the interpersonal encounter may have contributed to a reduction in the stigma felt by people who experience mental health problems. Gladwell (2005) identified that there are more complaints about poor communication by health care providers than any other aspect of health care intervention. It can therefore be concluded that good communication is a fundamental part of good nursing practice and contributes to good-quality care as evaluated by care recipients.

Reflection	
Identify at least three things that you have learned from this chapter.	1. 2. 3.
How do you plan to use this knowledge within clinical practice?	1. 2. 3.
How will you evaluate the effectiveness of your plan?	1. 2. 3.
What further knowledge and evidence do you need?	1. 2. 3.

SUMMARY
- Interpersonal skills and communication are key to establishing a therapeutic relationship.
- It is essential that nurses recognise the central importance of all aspects of communication within the therapeutic encounter.
- Trust is a fundamental component of the helping relationship.
- Caring involves enabling people to use their own resources for self care, not only providing care for the recipient.

FURTHER READING

Bonham, P. (2004) *Communicating as a mental health carer*. Cheltenham: Nelson Thornes

This book is geared towards first-year nursing students, and provides a comprehensive introduction to theories and skills of communication. The reader is guided through the text by thoughtful use of exercises and discussion points.

Donnelly, E. and Neville, L. (2008) *Communication and interpersonal skills*. Exeter: Reflect Press
This is an accessible text that introduces students to theories of communication, with exercises for students to self-assess their communication skills. It is targeted at nursing students on Common Foundation Programmes and uses exercises to develop understanding.

Freshwater, D. (ed.) (2002) *Therapeutic nursing: improving patient care through self awareness and reflection*. London: Sage
This book uses a reflective learning approach to explore the interpersonal process of patient care and the therapeutic encounter. It provides a particularly useful discussion of the development of self-awareness and personal skills.

Norman, I. and Ryrie, I. (eds) (2004) *The art and science of mental health nursing: a textbook of principles and practice*. Buckingham: Open University Press
This book provides a good introduction to a broad range of skills, topics and concepts to help the student to understand the contemporary context of mental health nursing practice. Despite its broad approach, it manages successfully to do justice to the topics and provides a balanced discussion of the therapeutic relationship and the nursing skills required to provide evidence-based practice.

Peplau, H.E. (1988) *Interpersonal relations in nursing* (2nd ed.). Basingstoke: Macmillan Education
This seminal work provides the reader with an enlightening discussion of Peplau's humanistic theory of practice. Basic principles are defined and the focus is on self-awareness and the helping relationship.

Chapter 4

Children, Family and Public Health

This chapter covers the following key issues:

- the practice and ethics of health promotion activity;
- the use of touch by the care giver;
- the concept of 'empathy';
- issues of lay/professional conflict;
- evaluating health promotion activities from the perspective of providers, payers, public and patients.

By the end of this chapter you should be able to:
- identify critical incidents from a case study;
- use Gibbs' reflective cycle to examine a critical incident;
- analyse the case study using frameworks of knowledge, identifying ethical issues and the importance of empathy in the caring process;
- consider how the knowledge of self impacts on the caring process using a theoretical framework;
- consider issues of lay professional conflict within health promotion activity;
- explore the use of touch in the caring relationship;
- consider how the care provided in this case study could be evaluated.

INTRODUCTION

The case study in this chapter reflects the work that may be undertaken by a nurse working in primary care and delivering the immunisation programme for children, but also recognising and acting to deliver broader health promotion interventions – in this case smoking cessation (**Essence of Care Benchmark – Promoting Health**).

The children, family and public health career pathway for nurses proposes that nurses will be intervening at a population level, including health needs assessment for populations, communities, groups, families and individuals. The childhood immunisation programme, led at population level by the Health Protection Agency (HPA *et al.*, 2005), and smoking cessation services, delivered by nurses working with individual families, are ways that nurses contribute to the maintenance and improvement of children and family health. This activity is partly a reflection of the recognition by health service policy-makers that, in order to sustain and 'afford' the NHS in the future, health professionals and society in general must ensure individuals engage in preserving their own health (Longley *et al.*, 2007). Within the New Labour policy library it was the document the *NHS Improvement Plan* (DH, 2004b) under the lead of the then Secretary of State for Health John Reid, which among its multitude of initiatives started to focus policy on 'greater concentration on better prevention rather than cure'. This focus has been emphasised by the publication of the White Paper *Choosing Health* (DH, 2004c) that focused on interventions for many of the public health 'time bombs' such as smoking and obesity.

Such policy directives impact on nursing care provision, as is seen in the proposal of community-based services in the policy document *Our Health, Our Care, Our Say* (DH, 2006a), which outlines plans for:

- shifting expenditure from hospitals to the community and preventative services;
- piloting a new NHS 'Life Check' (initially by questionnaire) to assess people's lifestyle risks, the right steps to take and provide referrals to specialists if needed.

It is moving the emphasis more towards enabling self-care (**ESC 2.iii; Essence of Care Benchmark – Principles of Self Care**).

- Supporting people to self-care by investment in the Expert Patient Programme, which is a series of educational programmes to enable the self-management of long-term conditions. These programmes are specifically designed to help individuals reduce the severity of symptoms and improve confidence, resourcefulness and self-efficacy (DH, 2001b).
- Developing an 'information prescription' for people with long-term health and social care needs and for their carers.
- Providing a Personal Health and Social Care Plan as part of an integrated health and social care record.
- Providing more support for carers including improved emergency respite arrangements.

THE CHILDREN, FAMILY AND PUBLIC HEALTH CASE STUDY

As a nurse working in a busy general practice in the middle of a city I was really pleased to be nominated to take forward the smoking cessation service in the practice. I took great pleasure in doing the local training and visiting the local health promotion library to get leaflets and some models that I could give out to the individual patients and show them the harm they are doing to their lungs by smoking. I put a lot of effort into putting up a display in the reception area and arranged the leaflets so that clients could help themselves.

One day when I was in the middle of baby clinic I noticed that there was a smell of cigarette smoke on a mum called Gemma bringing her three-month old baby in for immunisations. Once I had given the injection and advised Gemma accordingly I ventured to ask if she smoked. She answered quite defensively initially as if she was expecting me to be judgemental and ask her how she could put her baby's health at risk. When I said that I had been a smoker and had found it really difficult to give up, that in fact it took me about four attempts, she did seem to relax a little. I then asked her if she had ever tried to stop and said that she had managed to give up when she was pregnant but had started again as she found being at home with the baby very stressful and lonely. She insisted that she never smoked in front of the baby, although she found it hard to ask her mum and grandmother not to smoke when visiting or looking after her. When she had asked, her mum just replied that it is all a big nonsense and that her own grandmother smoked until she was 87 and never 'ailed' a day. Anyway if it is bad for your health all the tax you pay goes towards paying for the treatment you receive. That was something grandma had said when she was in hospital for the last time. She had all these machines hooked up to record her heart and breathing rate (she had had a heart attack) and joked at how much it all must cost. She joked that all the tax she had paid to the government through her 'cigs' was finally being spent on her needs!

When I asked her if she would like to try again to stop Gemma said she could use the money on other things and that her partner would be pleased with her if she did – he had also given up when she was pregnant but had not started smoking again. This was the frequent subject of arguing between them but Gemma felt it was unfair as he had been supported to stop by his workplace that had set up stop-smoking classes at the factory and even allowed attendance in work time. Her husband had also been supported by a group of friends who gave up together using the group at work. They were using the money they had saved to go on a boys' weekend away fishing.

We agreed that she would make an appointment to come and see me again if she wanted to give up and we could decide whether she should see me in a one-to-one or whether group meetings would be better. I gave her some written information on where else she could go for help if she decided not to return to me. I hope she does though as I felt we could establish a trusting relationship.

On leaving the room Gemma turned to me and said that she did not think she could stop but wanted to and didn't want to waste my time. I walked over to her, maintaining eye contact and put my hand on her arm and said that I understood that she may find it hard as a lot of people do, but that I would help her as much as I could and that there is lots of other help such as help lines, medications and even gum that she could try if will power was not enough alone. I flagged her notes to remind me to ask her again when she returned to the practice for the baby's next immunisations and will ensure the health visitor is updated in case she can offer further encouragement.

Critical incident analysis exercise

Using critical incident analysis as described at the end of Chapter 1, can you list all the elements from this case study that could be described as a critical incident? Include examples of practice that were either good or bad, as well as incidents that can give insight into practice, focusing specifically on why it was successful or could have been improved in some way. Give at least three positive examples and an example where the nurse could have improved the outcome for the service user.

Commentary on the case study

On the opposite page is a list of the possible critical incidents that could be used to reflect on within this case study and they have been mapped to the attributes and characteristics that service users valued in nurses as presented by Rush and Cook (2006) and Pryds-Jensen et al. (1993) as attributes of a 'caring nurse'.

Other possible critical incidents are:

- the revelation that her mum and grandmother smoke when visiting;
- probing to assess if she would like to try to stop smoking again;
- that Gemma felt her partner had an advantage as he had been supported to stop by his workplace that had set up stop-smoking classes and even allowed attendance in work time.

Possible critical incident	Commentary	Rush and Cook (2006) and Pryds-Jensen et al. (1993) attributes and characteristics.
The nurse undertook local training.	Important as a critical incident as this enables the nurse to undertake the interventions required with the necessary skills and knowledge and may increase confidence.	Competence. Knowledge. Practical skills. Self-confidence.
She used the local health promotion library to get leaflets for clients to hand out and for clients could help themselves.	Demonstrates her ability to use resources appropriately and access literature that includes interventions for clients in her care, which may enable health-promoting activity.	Competence. Communication. Demonstrate knowledge. Practical skills.
Used opportunistic approach to address health-promotion issue when she noticed that there was a smell of cigarette smoke on Gemma.	Very important as she used her assessment skills to judge the situation and decide to intervene when she realised Gemma was a smoker. She could easily have ignored the smell and continued with her busy clinic.	Demonstrates knowledge and competence. Self-confidence. Knowledge of others. Timing based on intuition. Committed. Honest. Demonstrate courage.
Addresses Gemma's defensive response and expectation of being judged by explaining that she had been a smoker and had found it really difficult to give up.	This demonstrated the nurse using intuition and experience to try to connect with Gemma and empathise with her situation.	Compassion. Kindness. Communication. Demonstrates knowledge. Self-confidence. Reflective self-knowledge. Knowledge of others. Demonstrate empathy. Timing based on intuition. Honest. Generous.
Gemma admitted that she found being at home with the baby very stressful and lonely.	This was a missed opportunity for intervention from the nurse. She could have explored further the networks Gemma has and opportunities for support such as referral into or existing contact with the HV service.	May have demonstrated a lack of knowledge re: health visiting (HV) services or support available for new mums and the incidence/implications of post-natal depression.
When Gemma was about to leave the nurse walked over to her, maintaining eye contact and put her hand on Gemma's arm saying that she understood that she may find it hard as a lot of people do but that she would help her as much as she could.	The response from the nurse here shows her commitment to helping Gemma, offering both compassion and information about some of the possible ways she can help her. This engenders trust and will be explored further later in this chapter.	Compassion. Kindness. Communication (use of touch). Self-confidence. Knowledge of others. Demonstrate empathy. Timing based on intuition. Committed.

Exercise using Gibbs' Reflective Cycle

Using Gibbs' reflective cycle (1988) (detailed in Chapter 1) to consider one of the critical incidents listed above or a different aspect of the case study, reflect further, working through each of the stages of the cycle and ensuring that you include what action you would take to improve user outcomes in the future. It may be the outcome for this particular user or replicating what has gone well for other care recipients.

Analysing the caring process using frameworks of knowledge

Working through a critical incident or using Gibbs' reflective cycle enables us to recognise how important it is to understand the knowledge that underpins an activity so that we can understand the way in which that knowledge is organised and applied in practice. In order to do this we will now explore the physical, cognitive and emotive domains of nursing and Carper's four fundamental patterns of knowing that underpin contemporary nursing practice.

Physical, cognitive and emotive domains or aspects

Activity

Can you think of examples of care given within this case study that fit within the:
- Physical domain?
- Cognitive domain?
- Emotive domain?

The physical domain

At first look this case study appears to have no relevant physical care delivered. However, physical care giving is not simply about performing a given task and should be considered in terms of holistic care delivery. The recognition of Gemma as a smoker, maintenance of eye contact and the therapeutic use of touch in order to reassure is akin to physical care giving (**ESC 6.ii**). That is, that physical care giving includes the application of knowledge, skills, values and attitudes within the physical act of doing for the patient (Allmark, 1998).

The cognitive domain

From the case study it is obvious that the nurse cares about the smoking cessation work she is undertaking. She sees value in it as expressed in her pleasure at being nominated to take forward the smoking cessation service in the practice. She also took 'great pleasure' in doing the local training and visiting the local health promotion library to get leaflets and some models to be used in the practice.

Activity

Why do you think she felt this way? Can you think of a professional reason and a personal motivation for her attitude?

The emotional domain

Activity

Having identified that the nurse has given up smoking herself and may feel committed to smoking cessation activity due to the negative impact on health of smoking, how do you think the nurse conveyed the fact that she cared about Gemma and wanted to help her to give up smoking within the case study?

Carper's *Fundamental Patterns of Knowing in Nursing*

Empirics

Empirics are the factual or science-based aspect of nursing. It involves describing, explaining and predicting phenomena. There are four levels of empirical knowing that are important in this case study. The first is the empirics of smoking itself.

The incidence
Around 10 million adults smoke cigarettes in Great Britain, which represents 23 per cent of men and 21 per cent of women (one-sixth of the population).

Smoking is highest among 20–24 year olds: 33 per cent of men and 29 per cent of women smoke.

Declines in smoking have been concentrated in older people. However, about half of all adults report that they have never smoked.

(Action on Smoking and Health (ASH), 2008)

The second is the empirics of the harm it does.

Risk of disease
Smoking causes almost 90 per cent of deaths from lung cancer, around 80 per cent of deaths from bronchitis and emphysema, and around 17 per cent of deaths from heart disease.

About one-third of all cancer deaths can be attributed to smoking. These include cancer of the lung, mouth, lip, throat, bladder, kidney, stomach, liver and cervix.

People who smoke between 1 and 14 cigarettes a day have eight times the risk of dying from lung cancer compared to non-smokers.

Smokers under the age of 40 have five times greater risk of a heart attack than non-smokers.

(Action on Smoking and Health (ASH), 2008)

The third is the empirics of the benefits of quitting.

Benefits of stopping smoking
Stopping smoking reduces the risk of developing many fatal diseases.

One year after stopping, the risk of a heart attack falls to about half that of a smoker and within 15 years falls to a level similar to that of a person who has never smoked.

Within 10–15 years of quitting, an ex-smoker's risk of developing lung cancer is only slightly greater than that of a non-smoker.

(Action on Smoking and Health (ASH), 2007)

The fourth is the empirics of the science around quitting.

Brief interventions in primary care
Brief interventions involve opportunistic advice, discussion, negotiation or encouragement. They are commonly used in many areas of health promotion by a range of primary and community care professionals.

For smoking cessation, brief interventions typically take between 5 and 10 minutes. The particular package that is provided will depend on a number of factors, including the individual's willingness to quit, how acceptable they find the intervention on offer and the previous

---

ways they have tried to quit. It may include one or more of the following:

- simple opportunistic advice to stop;
- an assessment of the patient's commitment to quit;
- an offer of pharmacotherapy and/or behavioural support;
- provision of self-help material and referral to more intensive support such as the NHS Stop Smoking Services.

(National Institute for Health and Clinical Excellence, 2006, p.5)

The empirics of smoking are expressed by the nurse through her competence gained in part through the attendance at a training course where she will have learned the facts and figures and also nursing interventions in order to promote successful quitting (**ESC 9.v; 9.vi**).

Aesthetics

The aesthetic of nursing involves not just the observation and description of a care recipient's behaviour and actions, but also an understanding of their view of what is significant in terms of needs and wants and experiences (**ESC 3.ii; 3.vi**). Empathy is an important concept in relation to the aesthetics of nursing, where the nurse is able to understand and appreciate the impact of an experience on another. To practise empathy is to maintain one's own identity while feeling with another, and is to be objective while at the same time offering support and understanding (Sitzer, 1996, p. 78). It has been defined as 'an affective state stemming from the apprehension of another's emotional state or condition' (Eisenburg and Miller, 1987) or an emotional response evoked by the affective state or situation of another person (Miller and Eisenburg, 1988). In their study of empathy and its relation to the occupational stress of nurses, Omdahl and O'Donnell (1999) argue that a health professional who experiences empathy is more likely to behave altruistically or intentionally for the benefit of the care recipient and so act with general concern for the individual and also communicate more effectively.

It is not necessary for the nurse to have personally experienced what the care recipient is going through – in this case recognising the need to quit smoking. There are, for example, many successful smoking-cessation advisers who have never smoked but can empathise with how difficult it is for individuals to quit. It is also likely that the nurse had experienced quitting very differently to Gemma in terms of context – she may not have been a new mum but had given up due to a recognition of the health impacts alone and individual factors – her family may have encouraged her to carry on smoking. There is also a danger that if the empathy is based on subjectively sharing the emotion of the care recipient, then the nurse will not be able to maintain their own identity and objectivity in the situation. This could lead both to poor care and advice and also emotional exhaustion or burnout (Omdahl and O'Donnell, 1999).

Activity

What type of understanding and application of skills and knowledge in this situation would have been different if the nurse had not been able to empathise as an ex-smoker? How would she have established empathy?

Ethics (the moral content of nursing knowledge)

Within the context of this case study the nurse is faced with the need to make a decision or choice relating to the detection of smoke on this mother's clothes. Carper's ethical dimension of knowing may help us to understand and resolve some of these dilemmas by providing the nurse with knowledge and insights into alternative courses of action with emphasis on the rights and dignity of the care recipient.

Activity

- Can you identify any ethical questions raised by the case study?
- Is it whether it is morally right or wrong to raise the issue of smoking in a consultation made specifically for another purpose?

This question could be asked of all opportunistic health promotion activity; activity that is aimed at increasing the awareness of the health effects of a specific activity, in this case smoking (Jones and Sidell, 1997). Is it therefore appropriate to intervene if the end is worth pursuing and is the intervention used by the nurse a legitimate influence for her to exercise over Gemma? Or is she interfering in the life of someone when she was not invited to do so formally as she was, for example, in immunising the baby?

Is the question rather of whether health gain and freedom of informed choice were the primary focus of the nurse's decision to intervene? Was the autonomy of the individual respected in order to bring out some benefit and did the intervention avoid harm? Avoiding harm is interesting in terms of the health professional's assumption that the harm to consider here is the harm to health of smoking.

So how do we understand why Gemma smokes? In Hilary Graham's research into the smoking activity undertaken by 'disadvantaged' women in the early 1990s she discovered that cigarettes provide a particularly crucial resource for those individuals who were facing difficult life events. Those, for example, facing parental illness and death and those living with financial hardship and under the threat of eviction described how cigarettes are viewed as a reliable friend in an uncertain and frightening world (Graham, 1993). Graham also identified how smoking was perceived to improve self-esteem and manage mood. In our case study Gemma may have been using the cigarettes for any one of these reasons.

Finally, the consequence of not intervening may need to be considered. Will there be an impact on the health of her child, herself and the likelihood of her partner starting to smoke again?

Activity

Consider the nurse's action in asking Gemma whether she smoked and offering her advice on quitting.
• Did she act in an ethical manner?

Personal knowledge

As a human activity, based on interpersonal and therapeutic relationships, personal knowledge is fundamental to good nursing practice, as this will impact on the nature and quality of the interpersonal relationships. It is about asking the question 'how do I know?'. Personal knowledge is thus concerned with an introspective awareness that allows the nurse to engage in the world of the care recipient, rather than being objectively detached from it, and to 'express an authentic, genuine self in interactions with others' (Freshwater, 2002).

Activity

How does the nurse engage with the world of the care recipient? What knowledge did she need to have about her self to allow her to do this successfully?

To explore this further it may be useful to look at the work of Davies and O'Berle (1990), work that referred particularly to the palliative care setting but is relevant to other care relationships. They identified elements of care including 'valuing, connecting, empowering, finding meaning, doing for and preserving integrity'.

'Valuing' is about respect and being non-judgemental (**ESC 3.vi; KSF Core dimension 6**). From the case study it was identified by the nurse that the care recipient was quite defensive about smoking. This may have been based on the pressure that she felt from her partner about giving up and the complexity of her situation in that her mother and grandmother were continuing to smoke even in front of the baby.

Activity

How did the nurse display respect for Gemma and avoid being judge-mental?

One very useful way of being non-judgemental and displaying respect could be thorough Davis and O'Berle's element of 'connecting', which is similar to empathising. It is about listening, understanding, having a caring attitude that says the person is important. Spending time and giving adequate time to care recipients is also an aspect of connecting.

Activity

The nurse in the case study worked in a busy practice and will have been in the middle of a busy immunisation clinic. How did she manage to give adequate time to Gemma (**ESC 17.ii**)?

There is significant evidence that to successfully quit smoking the individual needs to feel that they have made that decision and feel in control of the process – not forced and not bullied in any way – so, on one level, that is to 'self care'. This is about the nurse 'empowering' or 'enabling' Gemma to make her own decision. To do this she may ensure that she is fully informed about the decision to quit or continue smoking. One way of enabling this process is through finding 'meaning' in terms of what the individual's life is all about, which might involve spiritual assessment but, in this case study, is more about trying to understand the things that are driving Gemma to smoke and the things that may drive her to quit.

Activity

Make a list of all the things that might drive Gemma to continue smoking (for example, addiction) and another list of things that may drive her to quit (such as concerns regarding the health of her baby).

Davis and O'Berle also discuss the 'doing for' element of caring, which includes physical and emotional support and again is about negotiation and not taking over by, for example, giving Gemma the option of returning for smoking cessation advice if that is the option she wishes to take. 'Doing for' may also include referral on to a smoking-cessation group or to the health visitor who may be able to visit Gemma in her home to offer advice (**ESC 2.iii; 2.iv**).

Finally, the element of 'preserving integrity' is really about the nurse being able to avoid being incapacitated by the emotional effect of caring for another. In this case that may be succumbing to frustration or even anger if Gemma chose not to quit, or even a feeling of failure.

Activity

What empirical evidence may the nurse remind herself of if her attempt to encourage the individual to quit results in failure?

Lay–professional conflict

Each of us is an expert in our own health and notions of health are located within people's daily lives. Therefore, health and illness are complex sets of beliefs, which individuals develop from their understandings within their own social context. This may lead to conflicts with professional perceptions of health and illness (Nettleton, 2006).

Activity

Can you identify within the case study any examples of where lay–professional conflict occurred or may have occurred?

One of the most significant issues with health promotion activity of this kind is how the individual recipient views health itself. The nurse is promoting the view that Gemma can improve her health in that she can choose to smoke or not to smoke. However, we have already identified that there may be many complex drivers for Gemma continuing to smoke in terms of it being a support and, from the case study, we can add the experience of:

- her mum, who thinks quitting smoking is all a big nonsense;
- her mum's grandmother who smoked until she was 87 and never 'ailed' a day (until she had a heart attack and was hooked up to all sorts of

expensive equipment);
• the fact that even 'if it is bad for your health all the tax you pay goes towards paying for the treatment you receive'.

Theories of health promotion broadly identify five themes (Benner and Wrubel, 1989), three of which may be important here. The first sees health as the ability to fulfil social roles (Parsons, 1981) and may support the nurse's position in terms of the mother's ability to safely care for her child without exposing him to ill health. However, there are two flaws here. Gemma may feel that smoking helps to calms her nerves and fulfils a personal need in her that makes her better able to cope with motherhood. It ignores the person's sense of well-being, which can be improved by adopting medically risky behaviours. Also, in terms of immediacy, the impact of smoking cannot be immediately seen and recognised and so will not impact on the perception of fulfilling social role and function until the mum herself is in hospital when she is a grandma following a heart attack or the child develops asthma (which could, of course, be associated not with the smoking mum but the dampness of the house).

The second theme is health being viewed as a commodity. This is a technological and medicalised view and is reflected in the grandma's view that her tax is buying cures for her smoking-related illness and her belief that the technology to help her will be available.

Finally, health is viewed as a sense of coherence (Antonovsky, 1987) which emphasises the importance of belonging to a socio-cultural group in which its meanings are integrated and lived out as one's own concerns. Central to this is a belief of being in control. Within this model the belief that smoking helps Gemma's situation, in that it helps her relax or did not harm her grandma (and she was 87), is being slowly challenged by the health promotion activity of public policy. There is now a growing understanding and belief that smoking is harmful, as acknowledged by Gemma through her choice of not smoking in front of the baby. This understanding is creating a tension within Gemma's cultural group norms seen by the disagreement between the husband and his wife's family. In order to care for Gemma the nurse is presenting to her that her health is impacted by certain choices she makes, so that she can reappraise the situation she is in and seek help in order to quit smoking if that is her decision.

It is therefore important when undertaking health promotion activities in this scenario that the reasons for continuing smoking behaviours are understood within the individual's social context. Support that focuses on voluntary lifestyle behavioural change runs the risk of being seen as a victim-blaming approach, pathologising the individual's behaviour and failing to see the wider structural context (Bunton *et al.*, 1995).

The therapeutic relationship – the use of touch

Touch is a form of non-verbal communication influenced by the nurse's intentionality and a patient's perceptions of what is happening in a given situation. Experienced nurses reach an understanding of a care recipient's experience and possible responses to it through knowing the particular patient, the pattern of responses to date, the story portrayed and through using clinical knowledge (Benner *et al.*, 1996). This is gained through the experience of caring for many persons in similar situations, which sensitises the nurse to possible issues and concerns in particular situations. This experience enables the therapeutic relationship and motivates the nurse carer to undertake specific caring actions – one of which is touch (**KSF Core dimension 1 – Communication**).

While on one level it is very important to respect someone's personal space in order to maintain that individual's dignity and to display respect, touch can be an important tool in care provision. In the case study the use of touch is brief and could be considered of little consequence:

> I walked over to her, maintaining eye contact and put my hand on her arm and said that I understood that she may find it hard as a lot of people do, but that I would help her as much as I could . . .

Also touch in nursing is traditionally used to physically care or do something for a care recipient such as bathing or taking a blood pressure reading or pulse but it is also about the transference of feeling. Touch as a form of non-verbal communication can communicate comfort, security and warmth, having implications for emotional self-esteem. Expressive touch affects people's feelings of worth and self-esteem. Various studies (Tutton, 1991) identify how touch is a way of communicating caring and well-being, carries messages of acceptance, communicates trust and can be considered therapeutic. Many studies lend support to the experiences of nurses that touch has a comforting and calming effect upon a patient (Routosalo, 1999).

However, it is important to remember that the experience of touch varies between individuals depending on gender, age and, rather obviously, on the parts of the body touched. Touch is interpreted between individual participants according to their own subjective interpretive systems (Chang, 2001). Inappropriate touching, even when this is simply moving too close into someone's personal space, should be avoided (Edwards, 1998). In the case study, however, the use of touch is entirely appropriate and is used as an intervention modality in promoting comfort in a caring situation (Chang, 2001).

THE EVALUATION OF CARE

How can the impact of this care episode be measured? One way to consider the success of this care episode is to consider it from the perspective of providers, payers, public and patients, (Huycke and All, 2000) **(KSF Core dimension 4 – Service Improvement, and Core dimension 5 – Quality)**.

Providers

Providers, for example health care organisations, are interested in the process and outcomes including having the knowledge to deliver care and achieving the required health outcomes. Questions that might be asked include:

- was the nurse adequately trained to deliver the intervention?
- did the GP practice offer the appropriate levels of service, for example, if the mum chose to be referred to a smoking group how long would she have to wait until she got a place?
- was the nurse successful in persuading Gemma to try to quit smoking?

Payers

Payers are the general public in terms of taxpayers and they would be interested in the key measurables of affordability and access to care according to need. Questions asked may include:

- is there any evidence for this kind of opportunistic and brief intervention based on efficacy, i.e., does it work?
- did Gemma return for cessation advice and how many other individuals who were offered the same intervention or advice also tried to quit smoking (or were successful)?
- is the amount of time and effort being put into this smoking cessation intervention reaping benefits in terms of individual quitters?

Public

As a public service the care delivery must meet standards and regulation set by the government. This is achieved using the Healthcare Commission's *Standards for Better Health* (Healthcare Commission, 2004). The public therefore may seek information about whether the practice meets the Healthcare Commission's *Standards for Better Health* or is achieving good results in the National Patient Survey which is published online (**www.nhssurveys.org**).

Patients

Patients identify the characteristics of quality of care as:

- responsiveness;
- respect;
- timely response;
- confidence in performing procedures.

(Huycke and All, 2000)

Activity

How did the nurse measure up in this case study? Did she respond quickly to the situation and with respect? Was she confident in her approach? How do you know this?

Reflection	
Identify at least three things that you have learned from this chapter.	1. 2. 3.
How do you plan to use this knowledge within clinical practice?	1. 2. 3.
How will you evaluate the effectiveness of your plan?	1. 2. 3.
What further knowledge and evidence do you need?	1. 2. 3.

SUMMARY
- Health promotion is a fundamental component of nursing care in the twenty-first century.
- In order to practise health promotion ethically it is important to understand the perspective of the care recipient.
- Appropriate use of touch is fundamental to good nursing care.
- Empathy is an important concept in relation to the aesthetics of nursing, where the nurse is able to understand and appreciate the impact of an experience on another.
- It is important to acknowledge and understand issues of lay/ professional conflict in order to care for individual in a person-centred way.
- In order to quality-assure health promotion activity it is possible to explore outcomes from the perspective of providers, payers, public and patients.

FURTHER READING

Ewles, L. and Simnett, I. (2003) *Promoting health: a practical guide* (5th ed.). Edinburgh: Bailliere Tindall
Promoting health is an easy-to-read, practical guide for all those who practise health promotion in their everyday work. It provides a comprehensive and rigorous introduction to the theory and practice of health promotion, exploring concepts of health, health promotion and public health, discusses ethical issues, and maps out the agencies and people who play a part. It also looks at assessing health promotion needs, and researching, planning and evaluating health promotion work, and focuses on 'hands on' health promotion, such as how to help people to change their health behaviour.

McMahon, P. and Pearson, A. (1998) *Nursing as therapy*. London: Chapman and Hall
This book includes material on quality, practice and the politics of nursing; and examines therapeutic nursing as the centre of health care delivery. It contains critical challenges to nurses, which will help to enhance professional practice.

Naidoo, J. and Wills, J. (2005) *Public health and health promotion: developing practice*. Edinburgh: Bailiere Tindall
The focus of this book is on dilemmas and challenges which underpin health promotion – where is the evidence and how is health promotion practice informed by it. The book includes a wide range of case study

material reflecting the diversity of health promotion practice. All case studies are accompanied by commentaries from the authors, allowing the reader to see the relevance to their own practice.

Nettleton, S. (2006) *The sociology of health and illness* (2nd ed.). Cambridge: Polity Press
The central theme of this book is the notion that we are moving towards a new paradigm of health and health care in which people are no longer passive recipients of treatment when they are 'ill' but active participants in the maintenance of their own health. This reflects the current health policy of health promotion, health care in the community and choice.

Routasalo, P. (1999) 'Physical touch in nursing studies: a literature review'. *Journal of Advanced Nursing*, 30(4): 843–50
This article gives a broad overview of the literature surrounding the use of touch in nursing contexts.

Chapter 5

First Contact, Access and Urgent Care

The key issues that will be addressed in this chapter are:

- the importance of respect for the individual including privacy;
- the importance of enabling understanding and empowerment through timely information giving;
- the value of the appropriate use of humour;
- the importance of underpinning the technically safe environment with compassionate and respectful care;
- the role of multi-agency or interdisciplinary working to enable the smooth transition of the care recipient's journey through the health care system;
- the role of user articulation in enhancing the quality of health care service provision.

By the end of the chapter you will be able to:

- identify critical incidents from a case study;
- use Gibbs' reflective cycle to examine a critical incident;
- analyse the case study using frameworks of knowledge to identify relevant issues in the care of people with urgent care needs;
- analyse the case study using frameworks of knowledge identifying ethical issues and the importance of user articulation in the caring process;
- explore the use of humour in the caring relationship;
- consider how the care provided in this case study could be evaluated.

INTRODUCTION

The case study in this chapter explores the experience of a female admitted to hospital via the accident and emergency department, unable to pass urine and in a lot of discomfort (**Essence of Care Benchmark – Continence and Bladder and Bowel Care**). It is explored through the care recipient articulating her experiences through a letter of complaint to the hospital.

While the rights and views of those accessing NHS services were strengthened through the Conservative government's introduction of the *Patient's Charter* in 1991 (DH, 1991a) it was *The New NHS: Modern, Dependable* (DH, 1997) and *The NHS Plan* (DH, 2000) that started to articulate the quality benchmarks that care recipients in the NHS should expect during care episodes. Indeed, the standardisation of complaints and compliments policy through the NHS expected by the Healthcare Commission *Standards for Better Health* (HCC, 2004) set out a process through which individuals were encouraged to articulate both their positive and negative experiences, and established an expectation that NHS Trusts respond to care recipients by exploring the causes of such situations and putting into place actions to prevent them happening again.

The nurses caring for the care recipient in this case study are trained to respond to a variety of undifferentiated needs and may be caring for individuals of all ages, enabling them to manage their own health care through advice, information or treatment for illness or disturbances in mental health and well-being. That is, in the first contact, access and urgent care pathways. The issues raised by the care recipient refer to breakdowns in the organisation of care, failure by some members of the team to recognise her specific need for 'care' in the physical, cognitive and emotion domains and the comfort received from one skilled member of staff who successfully 'cared' for her when removing her catheter.

THE FIRST CONTACT, ACCESS AND URGENT CARE CASE STUDY

To whom it may concern

I was recently admitted to Ward 73 via the Accident and Emergency Department, as I had acute retention of urine, necessitating catheterisation. Unfortunately, I experienced poor care in both A&E and on the ward, and wanted to raise a number of concerns with you.

1. When I saw my GP, she decided that I needed admission and phoned through to the duty doctor from urology to arrange my admission via the Accident and Emergency Department. However, when I arrived, nobody seemed to be expecting me. The triage nurse asked me a number of what I would consider intimate questions, which I found very embarrassing, particularly as a group of youths were sniggering nearby. I was then left sitting in the waiting room, while the triage nurse went to see what was happening. By this time, I was in acute discomfort, feeling dizzy and nauseous and found it not only very uncomfortable to be sitting in a hard plastic chair, but also felt very vulnerable and alone.

2. After some time, I was taken through to a cubicle, and told that the urologist was on his way to see me. I had been unable to contact anyone to accompany me to the hospital, so once again was left on my own. By now I was in considerable pain. I was not offered any pain relief or any explanation as to why it might not be appropriate. I appreciate that the nursing staff in Accident and Emergency must be extremely busy, but would have appreciated a few words of kindness, instead of being left to feel as though I was in the way.

3. The urologist came to see me, and after asking some questions, washing his hands and feeling my tummy he catheterised me, which at least had the effect of alleviating the pain. The nurse who acted as chaperone during the catheterisation paid little attention to me and, instead, seemed more interested in discussing a recent social event with the doctor. I would have preferred to be seen by a lady doctor but he seemed to know what he was doing and I hardly felt a thing when he catheterised me.

4. The urologist informed me that he would need to admit me, as he thought I might have a stricture in my urethra and he wanted to run some further investigations before sending me home. He explained what a stricture was and was very reassuring that he would be able to sort the problem out for me. There were no available beds on the urology ward, so a bed elsewhere needed to found. This was at approx. 11 p.m. The nurse went to arrange my admission, saying that she would be back in a while. At about 1 a.m., I was still waiting to be admitted, having been left for much of that time on my own. I buzzed for a nurse a couple of times, only to be told that they were still trying to find me a bed. When I buzzed at 2 a.m., the nurse came to see me and expressed surprise that I was still there. She told me that a bed had been found on the dermatology ward and she would arrange for me to be taken there.

5. On arrival at the ward a staff nurse met me and took me to the prepared bed and said that she would be back to admit me. She came back a few minutes later and proceeded to fill in some paper work (**Essence of Care Benchmark – Record Keeping; ESC 6.iii**). At no time did she introduce herself to me or show any interest in anything, other than filling in the answers to the questions that she was required to address. No other nurse introduced themselves to me during my brief stay on the ward and I was left feeling that they had little interest or understanding of my condition or well-being.

6. The next morning, the urologist came to see me and decided that the catheter could be removed and that, if I was passing urine freely, I could be discharged and come back to outpatients for the tests. I was very worried about the catheter being removed but the nurse who came to see me this time was very efficient and did not hurt me at all. She spoke to me during the whole procedure explaining what she was doing, what it might feel like and distracting me with little jokes (**ESC 3.iv**). The first time I needed to pass urine, I asked a nurse if I needed to measure my urine and, if so, could she find me a jug or other receptacle. She informed me that she was not my named nurse who was responsible for my care and would find some-one to help me. Some 20 minutes later, I managed to get a jug to pass urine into, and left it in the female toilets, with my name written on a paper towel under the jug. I did the same thing three more times throughout the day, letting a nurse know what I had done. When I left the ward to go home, all four jugs of urine were still on the window sill where I left them, so I presume that my fluid balance chart had not been filled in either (**ESC 27.ii; 29.ii; 29.iii**) (I used to be a nurse, and therefore am aware of the impor-tance of such measurements in situations like mine).

I would not usually complain, but felt that the care that I received was largely inadequate, and it left me feeling distressed and angry. I hope that no one else ever finds themselves in this situation.

I look forward to hearing from you.

Critical incident analysis exercise

Using critical incident analysis, can you list all the elements from this case study that could be described as a critical incident? You may wish to refer to the work of Benner (1984) detailed in Chapter 1, but particularly think about incidents:

- in which the nurse's intervention made a difference to the care recipi-ent;
- that led to a breakdown of some kind.

Commentary on the case study

The following is a list of the possible critical incidents in this case study that could be used for reflection and they have been mapped to the attributes and characteristics that service users valued in nurses as presented by Rush and Cook (2006) and Pryds-Jensen *et al.* (1993) as attributes of a 'caring nurse'.

Possible critical incident	Commentary	Rush and Cook (2006) and Pryds-Jensen *et al.* (1993) attributes and characteristics.
The triage nurse asked 'a number of intimate questions' in the waiting room in front of a group of 'sniggering' youths.	This showed disregard for the privacy or comfort of the care recipient who, while suffering physical pain, also felt humiliated at having such an experience in public.	While the nurse may have been technically competent in terms of the triage assessment she failed to show: Compassion. Reflective self-knowledge. Knowledge of others. Empathy. She was not concerned to act on the basis of ethical values and attitudes in terms of protecting the privacy and dignity of the individual.
The lady stated that 'I appreciate that the nursing staff in Accident and Emergency must be extremely busy, but would have appreciated a few words of kindness, instead of being left to feel as though I was in the way'.	Again, while in pain she was led to feel isolated and it is almost as if she felt guilty for causing the staff extra work. A simple acknowledgement and apology for the wait may have helped her to feel reassured.	Again, the staff failed to show: Compassion. Reflective self-knowledge. Knowledge of others. Empathy. And they were not concerned to act on the basis of ethical values and attitudes.
On arrival the urologist catheterised her, which alleviated the pain. Although she would have preferred a woman he seemed to know what he was doing and she hardly felt a thing.	This is an example of physical care giving by a technically competent practitioner (**ESC 22.ii**). While it is not always possible to provide same sex carers it might have been possible for one of the female nurses to undertake the catheterisation procedure. If this was not possible, an explanation may have reassured her.	This shows the attributes of: Competence. Knowledge. Practical skills. But perhaps a lack of: Communication. Knowledge of others or empathy.
Despite being very worried about the catheter being removed, the nurse who came to see me this time was very efficient and did not hurt me at all. She spoke to me during the whole procedure explaining what she was doing, what it might feel like and distracting me with little jokes.	This critical incident is a good example of care giving by someone who is competent in the physical, cognitive and emotional domains and takes time to reassure and 'care' for the care recipient.	It demonstrates: Competence. Knowledge. Kindness. Communication. She has self-confidence and her use of humour shows timing based on intuition and creativity in distracting the individual from a potentially uncomfortable procedure. She approaches the patient with a positive attitude and acts calmly to control stressful situations.
When I asked for help one nurse informed me that she was not the named nurse who was responsible for my care, and would find someone to help me and I waited in discomfort for 20 minutes before managing to get a jug to pass urine into.	Subdividing the nursing teams and delegating individual patients to specific nurses is one way of organising care delivery on a ward and can work very successfully. However, this nurse may have shown lack of commitment by not helping the individual. Alternatively, she may simply have not known how to care for her, been in the middle of a different and urgent episode of care or been unable to find a member of staff who could help.	Regardless of the reason why this nurse was unable to help the individual, she demonstrates lack of communication skills, knowledge or compassion in recognising the care recipient was in discomfort.

Other possible critical incidents include the following.

- Once moved to the cubicle she was again left on her own in considerable pain. No pain relief or any explanation as to why it might not be appropriate was given.
- The nurse who acted as chaperone during the catheterisation paid little attention to her and, instead of comforting her, discussed a recent social event with the doctor.
- There were no available beds on the urology ward and she waited three hours for a bed on dermatology (**ESC 13.i**).
- The admitting nurse on dermatology did not introduce herself or show any interest in anything other than filling in the answers to the questions that she was required to address. No other nurse introduced themselves to her during her brief stay on the ward. She was left feeling that the dermatology ward nurses had little interest or understanding of her condition or well-being.
- When she left the ward to go home, all four jugs of urine she had passed were still on the window sill, unmeasured.

Exercise using Gibbs' Reflective Cycle

Using Gibbs' reflective cycle (1988) (detailed in Chapter 1) to consider one of the critical incidents listed above or a different aspect of the case study, reflect further on the case study by working through each of the stages of the cycle, ensuring that you include the action you would take to improve user outcomes in the future. It may be an improved outcome for this particular user, improving care giving for future care recipients or replicating what has gone well for other care recipients.

Analysing the caring process using frameworks of knowledge

Working through a critical incident or using Gibbs' reflective cycle enables us to recognise how important it is to understand the knowledge that underpins an activity so that we can understand the way in which that knowledge is organised and applied in practice. In order to do this we will explore the physical, cognitive and emotive domains of nursing and Carper's four fundamental patterns of knowing that underpin contemporary nursing practice.

Physical, cognitive and emotive domains or aspects

Activity

Can you think of examples of care given within this case study that fit within the
- Physical domain?
- Cognitive domain?
- Emotive domain?

The physical domain

In this case study physical care giving was a priority, once the care recipient was seen by the urologist. This is demonstrated in terms of the catheterisation to relieve her symptoms of pain. It was likely that hospital policy determined that a consultant urologist performed this procedure due to the unknown cause of retention and, therefore, the possible complications of the procedure.

Competency is seen as the ability of an individual care giver that is required for a particular role or post (Manley and Garbett, 1998) and is the application of skills and knowledge, but competency involves more than performing a given task. It also involves cognitive, psychomotor and affective domains (Curzon, 1990) but, in the case of technical competency, it is about the urologist having the skill sets required to undertake the given role (i.e. catheterisation of an individual with unknown cause of retention of urine). It could be argued here that the care recipient should have been catheterised sooner in order to relieve her pain but if, on attempting catheterisation, a less competent individual, in this case the staff nurse, had faced unseen complications due to the unknown cause of retention and therefore acted both outside hospital policy and outside her scope of practice (NMC, 2008), she would not have been acting in the best interest of the individual.

The cognitive domain

When facing illness, whether it is curable or not (or indeed any stressful life experience), it can be normal for the individual to question why this is happening. One of these questions might be about the cause of any suffering experienced (Fredriksson, 1999) and result in an attempt to rationalise the situation. It is also a human trait to practise defensive reasoning (Argyris, 1991); that is, to rationalise about a situation so that the understanding of it does not conflict with personally held beliefs or need (**ESC 3.vi**). As a person who has worked as a nurse, the care recipient will have entered A&E with personal beliefs about the care she would receive. She may have expected immediate assessment as her GP had phoned the department and so they were expecting her arrival, and she may have expected that they would prioritise her pain relief. When this did not happen it appears that she rationalised the situation in order to understand it within a context that did not damage her belief in the quality of care she would receive. She rationalises that her treatment was lacking because she 'appreciate(s) that the nursing staff in Accident and Emergency must be extremely busy'.

Activity

How could the nursing staff have enabled her to rationalise the situation more clearly by understanding her cognitive care needs?

Information giving would have been a way to enable her to understand her wait and rationalise it more productively (**ESC 6**). Often people can be reassured simply by explaining the reason for the wait and the approximate expected waiting time. This is one explanation of the signs now seen in A&E and outpatient department giving approximate waiting times and the cause such as 'the department is experiencing a high volume of patients'.

The emotional domain

When considering the cognitive domain it is also apparent that the search for reason or explanation where there is no clear-cut answer leaves the care recipient needing emotional support or a 'partner' who is willing to listen and help in the struggle to understand. Such reinforcement of 'being' relates to the human desire for meaning and love (Fagerström et al., 1998) that, in a situation such as that described in the case study, can be translated to a need simply to be 'seen', to have her immediate needs acknowledged and be reassured that she is and will be 'cared for', both in the physical and emotional domain.

Carper's *Fundamental Patterns of Knowing in Nursing*

Empirics

Empirics are the factual or science-based aspects of nursing. This involves describing, explaining and predicting phenomena. Empirics can be related to the organisation of care and, in the instance of this case study, what was known about the admission of the care recipient to A&E, her known diagnosis and the required intervention.

Using empirics it is possible to argue that the department did not care for this lady adequately because they knew she was coming (her GP had referred her verbally) but that, on her arrival, they appeared 'not to be expecting her', so there must have been a breakdown in communication somewhere. Treating this as a critical incident may reveal where the breakdown occurred. Was it between the GP and the department, i.e. the referral call was not made? Did the person who received the referral forget to inform the department of her imminent arrival, was the form put on the 'wrong' pile, or was the department simply too busy to prepare for her? All of these issues may have possible solutions, whether it be reviewing and improving referral mechanisms or introducing more effective triage procedures so individuals in pain are seen as a priority (**ESC 2; KSF Core dimension 1; ESC 17.i**).

Activity

Can you think of any other information that the department knew about the lady on arrival that could have improved her care?

Aesthetics

The aesthetic of nursing involves not just the observation and description of a care recipient's behaviour and actions, but also an understanding of their view of what is significant in terms of needs and wants and experiences. To explore this further it may be useful to look at the types of caring needs that have been described in the work of Fagerström *et al.* (1998). These are goal-oriented needs based on scientific knowledge of medicine and then the specifically human needs that require fulfilment for the well-being of people, reducing pain and enhancing well-being. These 'human' needs include:

- belonging to a loving environment;
- education in living within human communion;
- the possibilities of receiving and giving proof of friendship and tenderness;
- the longing for confirming relationships as the primacy;
- the deepest desire of humans is for life, love and meaning.

In her letter the care recipient describes two very different experiences: one in A&E where she stated that 'I...would have appreciated a few

words of kindness, instead of being left to feel as though I was in the way';
and then the experience of having her catheter removed when the nurse
was 'very efficient and did not hurt me at all. She spoke to me during the
whole procedure explaining what she was doing, what it might feel like
and distracting me with little jokes.' The difference between the two
episodes demonstrates how different care episodes felt to a recipient –
one nurse engages in caring for the individual's 'human caring needs' and
one where these needs are simply ignored (**ESC 5.i; 5.iii**). It is the difference between what Fagerström *et al.* (1998) refer to as the 'satisfied
patient', who feels confident in the nurse's knowledge and skills and
feels taken care of, noticed and well looked after. This creates a sense
of well-being and comfort and is enabled by the care recipient feeling their
wishes are acknowledged and the nurse's way of relating to them being
friendly, pleasant and encouraging. This is opposed to the 'complaining
and dissatisfied patient' (Fagerström *et al.*, 1998), who is anxious and
uncertain because of the lack of clear diagnosis or the experience of
pain and who is therefore searching for security and reassurance. If this
is not forthcoming due to lack of guidance or communication, the need
for security or reassurance is not fulfilled.

Activity

Give two or three examples of how the nurse in A&E could have enabled
the care recipient to feel more cared for and satisfied.

Ethics

Within the context of this case study one of the issues that could be
explored within an ethical frame is the question of whether it was morally
justifiable for the ward nurse not to offer help as she was not the care
recipient's named nurse. This is a scenario that may be played out in
different ways in care settings with a nurse who is busy with a different
patient or distracted and therefore failing to respond to the care needs
requested. To act ethically is a process of deliberation in a specific situation (Johns, 1995) and the application of ethical principles may be a
starting point: did the nurse's response affect the patient's autonomy or
the right of the care recipient to make their own decisions and direct their
life? What attention did the nurse pay to the principle of beneficence – the
responsibility of doing good and so providing benefit or beneficial treat-
ment/care to the person? Did she avoid non-maleficence – the
responsibility of avoiding harm to the person and did she adhere to the
principle of justice, the responsibility to be equitable and fair in the way
we treat others (**ESC 9**)?

However, the dilemma with taking such an approach is that it simply is not clear what the answers to these questions are. Yes, there was potential harm in that the care recipient was in some discomfort in not being able to find a jug to urinate into, but would there be long-term harm – could she go back into retention, for example? In terms of beneficence, where did the nurse's responsibility to the patient start and end? Should her named nurse have provided a jug before in anticipation of the need to urinate? In terms of equity, would the patients for whom she was named nurse suffer if she was to help this particular care recipient?

There is therefore a tension between ethical principles and the situational ethics (Cooper, 1991) and it is important to ask whether conflicts exist between the values used in the situation and those that may have been employed by others, i.e., given the same situation would other nurses have acted in the same way? Situational ethics can be classified based on levels of conflicting values within experience (Johns, 1995). The first level is within situations of conflicting value within the nurse. The second level is conflicting values between the nurse and the patient (which can include situations of conflicting values within the patient and between the patient and their families), and situations of conflicting values between the nurse and other nurses/health care workers, acknowledging the organisational context of practice. In the organisational context of the ward with this 'outlier' from urology, were the expectations of the organisation of the nurses in terms of being able to care for her adequately, unfounded? Was the staffing on the ward at such a level that the nurses simply could not deliver a reasonable level of care?

Personal knowledge

As a human activity, based on interpersonal and therapeutic relationships, personal knowledge is fundamental to good nursing practice, as this will impact on the nature and quality of the interpersonal relationships. Again, using the example of the nurse who failed to help the care recipient as she was not her named nurse, it may be that the nurse involved was trying to protect herself from the stress of being involved in another person's care: trying in some way to protect herself from the further anxiety and sustain herself through yet another unmanageable shift due to an impossible workload. This 'burnout' avoidance may be a symptom of the inadequacy of the system in which the nurse is working. The failure does not lie with the individual nurses but with a system that fails to develop and sustain caring practices (Benner and Wrubel, 1989). This will be explored in further detail in Chapter 8.

User articulation

As briefly discussed in the introduction to this chapter, one of the policy directives outlined by the Labour government has been the introduction of quality benchmarks, one of which is the NHS ability to demonstrate its response to feedback by care recipients (**ESC 12.i; 12.ii**). This is under-pinned by the policy direction towards a patient-led NHS as set out in the policy document *Creating a Patient led NHS* (DH, 2005b). On a strategic level the government is moving the NHS towards a model of service delivery that is led by the patients it will care for. This can be achieved through responding to complaints but also by involving service users at every level of the organisation including NHS boards being chaired by lay members. While strategically the NHS movement towards a patient-led organisation is fraught with difficulties, on an individual level the question of how we allow care recipients to lead their care experience needs to be asked. The importance of having a voice within that caring relationship is vital (DH, 2000). However, questions need to be asked about what we mean by user involvement. User involvement can encompass a number of different strategies as detailed below.

Level of involvement	Methods	Tasks
Informed	Newsletters, leaflets, posters, radio	Informing patients about entitlements, resources, new services, etc.
Consultation	Focus or discussion groups, semi-structured interviews, questionnaires	Finding out about patient views of services
Collaboration/partnership	Committees, working groups	Agreeing priorities for service improvements
User control	Self-help and support groups, user groups	Users decide priorities and action in response to need

(Tanner and Harris, 2008)

The concept of empowerment should also be considered. Empowerment is concerned with the structure of the power relationship between users and providers of care, and the level of involvement in decisions about health care reflects the degree of empowerment of care recipients. See Figure 1 on page 92.

The therapeutic relationship – the use of humour

Theories concerning the use of humour in health care can be seen to look at the direct and indirect effects of humour (McCreaddie and Wiggins,

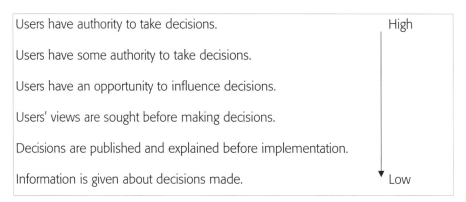

Figure 1 Degrees of empowerment (Brager and Specht, 1973)

2008). The direct effects include the theory that humour in terms of laughter creates physiological changes in the body, which are positive and conducive to health, or that humour and/or laughter may create a positive emotional state that creates health benefits. A good example of this would be that appropriate use of humour may reduce the experience of pain.

The indirect effects of humour may be in moderating the adverse effects of stress via the individual's cognitive perception, thereby enhancing the ability to cope and negating the known negative physical effects of stress. Also that humour is known to have a number of potential benefits in relation to interpersonal skills or social support. However, the literature surrounding these assertions regarding the direct and indirect effects of humour shows that the research is not conclusive (McCreaddie and Wiggins, 2008).

Martin (2006) views the use of humour in terms of regulating emotions to produce coping and Wooten (1992) sees the use of humour also being task-based in that it enables 'getting the job done'. Humour is certainly a means of providing distraction and this is how it was used within the case study. While it is important to acknowledge that there may be times when humour is not appropriate, creating humour exclusion zones (for example within a care area or by a profession) would fail to recognise shared commonalities and understandings between patients and nurses (McCreaddie and Wiggins, 2008) which are key to establishing a therapeutic relationship.

THE EVALUATION OF CARE

How can the impact of this care episode be measured? It can be understood in light of two conditions, the resource structure of the care organisation and the patient's preferences (Wilde Larsson and Larsson, 1999). The evaluation may therefore include assessment of the following.

1. Medical technical competence of the care givers – the ability of the care giver to perform physical care in a safe and competent manner. This may include questions about the competency of the urologist but also about the length of time taken for a competent individual to be available to catheterise. Was it appropriate to have to wait for the urologist? Could a member of the nursing staff have performed the catheterisation? Issues over appropriate pain relief could also be questioned. Could pain relief have been given on admission following triage?

2. The physical-technical conditions of the care organisation – having the right environment and equipment in order to facilitate care delivery. Questions could be asked here about the unpreparedness of the A&E department to receive the care recipient, the provision of a comfortable waiting area and privacy when being assessed. Why was the care recipient not moved to a private room to be assessed? In terms of the admission onto a ward, the big issue is whether admission to a ward that did not specialise in urology was appropriate.

3. The degree of identity orientation in the attitude and actions of the care givers. Did the individual feel that she was treated with dignity and with respect by the nurses at all times? Several of the points included in the care recipient's letter refer to where she felt she had been let down in this respect. One example is when she was being catheterised by the urologist and the nurse was 'more interested in discussing a recent social event with the doctor'.

Activity

What would have been more appropriate care for the nurse to undertake while chaperoning the urologist on this occasion?

4. The socio-cultural atmosphere of the care organisation could be assessed by asking whether the organisation restricted the desires and needs of the care recipient. Again, the articulation of her experience indicates that the care recipient did not feel that her needs and desires were provided for. One question in this regard is to ask whether she was able to maintain her dignity at all times. Possible evidence to the contrary is the incident when youths snigger at her during the triage process.

Reflection	
Identify at least three things that you have learned from this chapter.	1. 2. 3.
How do you plan to use this knowledge within clinical practice?	1. 2. 3.
How will you evaluate the effectiveness of your plan?	1. 2. 3.
What further knowledge and evidence do you need?	1. 2. 3.

SUMMARY

- Respecting an individual's privacy and need for information can help to alleviate stress and suffering associated with an acute episode of illness.
- While care recipients need and value technically competent care, it is vital that this is underpinned by care that acknowledges their need to be respected and treated as individuals.
- The organisational systems that facilitate inter-professional working are essential to ensure team working and enable the care recipient's efficient and effective journey through the health care system.
- User articulation is a right for all care recipients and is a powerful evaluative tool that can be used to enhance the quality of health care service provision.

FURTHER READING AND RESOURCES

Benner, P. and Wrubel, J. (1989) *The primacy of caring*. New York: Addison Wesley
This book gives first-person accounts from practising nurses which

provide students with expert role models to understand how caring makes a critical difference for patients and their families.

Department of Health (2005) *Now I feel tall.* London, HMSO
Aimed at chief executives, directors and all staff who deliver the National Health Service, this DH document is designed to make the NHS more aware of the importance of improving patients' emotional experience and the relevance of this to creating a patient-led NHS. It identifies the drivers improving patients' emotional experience, gives examples of how this has been achieved by organisations across the NHS, and makes at times quite inspirational reading.

Gerry Robinson and Daniel Barry (2007) *Can Gerry Robinson Fix The NHS?* DVD, Open University
This DVD contains the three programmes from the television series that follows Sir Gerry Robinson, businessman and management consultant, in his mission to reduce waiting lists at Rotherham General Hospital within six months and with no money. It looks at the use of performance management techniques, use of resources and the culture and attitudes of the clinical staff.

Richardson, R. (ed.) (2008) *Clinical skills for student nurses: theory, practice and reflection.* Exeter: Reflect Press
This textbook has been compiled for pre-registration students to include the essential procedures needed to meet the competencies of the Essential Skills Clusters (NMC, 2007). It presents up-to-date evidence-based clinical skills, enabling student nurses to deliver clinically effective patient-focused care and provides evidence for procedures related to every aspect of a person's care.

Chapter 6

Acute and Critical Care and Cultural Competency

The key issues that will be addressed in this chapter are:

- the importance of cultural competency in care delivery;
- respecting the expertise and the involvement of parents and informal carers in the formal caring context;
- the concept of kindness and its meaning in health care contexts;
- the ethical requirement for informed consent in health care contexts;
- the provision of holistic care which recognises the importance of spiritual and cultural belief systems.

By the end of the chapter you will be able to:
- identify critical incidents from a case study;
- use Gibbs' reflective cycle to examine a critical incident;
- analyse the case study using frameworks of knowledge to identify relevant issues in the care of people with acute and critical illness;
- consider the importance of informed consent in the caring process;
- consider issues of cultural competency within health care provision;
- explore the meaning of kindness in the caring relationship;
- consider how the care provided in this case study could be evaluated.

INTRODUCTION

Providing unscheduled or emergency care for individuals of all ages with various clinical, technical or nursing needs, and in situations that are quite often life threatening, can be very stressful and requires health professionals to possess skill and competence with the ability to remain calm. The case study in this chapter illustrates a care episode seen through the eyes of the father of a boy admitted via the accident and emergency department with acute appendicitis. Without immediate surgical intervention there is a significant risk that the appendix will perforate, leading to peritonitis, which is potentially life threatening. This stressful situation is potentially heightened as the parents have only been resident in the United Kingdom (UK) for four years and they acknowledge in the letter the difficulties of having English as a second language. Despite this the father is so impressed with the care received that he writes to the matron describing the quality of the care they experienced as a family. He refers to kindness, information giving and involvement in the care of his son as the reasons for his compliments, describing the NHS as a first-class service.

The UK today is a 'multicultural, multi ethnic and multiple language society' (Meddings and Haith-Cooper, 2008). The case study explores the issue of, and demonstrates examples of, the provision of culturally competent care. It challenges you to explore the ways in which you, as a care giver, can provide appropriate care to individuals whose ethnic, cultural and language backgrounds are different to your own (**ESC 4.i; 9.i; KSF Core dimension 6 – Equality and Diversity**).

THE ACUTE AND CRITICAL CARE AND CULTURAL COMPETENCY CASE STUDY

Dear Matron

I am writing to express my sincere gratitude for the care that my six-year-old son Masood received when he was on Ward 4 recently. He was admitted via the Accident and Emergency Department with acute appendicitis, and was rushed straight to theatre before being admitted to the ward. As you can imagine, it was a very anxious time for us all, including our other son, Hakim, who is 8, although he was at home with his grandmother when Masood was admitted through casualty.

I cannot fault the care that Masood received. We were greeted by a nurse as we entered the casualty and taken straight through to a room, where the doctor came and examined Masood and explained that he probably had appendicitis, but that he was going to get a surgeon to come and see him. He started a drip, and the nurse, who accompanied him, was very good, making sure that Masood knew exactly what was happening, and she kept him occupied so that he did not focus on the needle going into his arm. He also asked our permission to give Masood some pain relief and of course we gave our permission. The nurse explained that the pain relief and something to stop Masood feeling sick would be injected through the drip, to avoid having to give him another injection.

We arrived in the UK from Iran four years ago and although my wife speaks and understands English quite well, she sometimes struggles to understand complex terms. The nurse made sure that we fully understood what the doctor had told us, and told us to ask any questions that we had at any time. She said that if she was unable to address them, she would make sure she either found out for us, or would get someone else to come and talk to us.

The surgeon came to see Masood and decided that he needed to go straight to theatre before the appendix burst, leading to further complications. He asked us to sign a consent form. Again, the nurse ensured that we fully understood what we were signing and what was going to happen to Masood. She then invited my wife to help to prepare Masood for theatre, saying that this would help him to feel more relaxed. When it was time to go to theatre, she said that we could accompany him up to the theatre and my wife could stay with him until he was asleep.

When Masood was asleep, the theatre nurse said that they would look after him, and we would be able to see him very soon. The nurse, who had accompanied us from casualty, then took us to the ward where Masood would go after theatre. When his operation was over, a ward nurse asked my wife if she wanted to go with him to collect Masood. In the theatre room, he was quite distressed, although the theatre nurse did explain that he had had painkillers. She suggested that my wife might want to climb onto the trolley with Masood, so that she could cuddle him and give him comfort. Although he was still obviously in pain, he did settle when my wife did this and she felt that she was doing something to help to alleviate our son's distress.

On the ward, the nurses were very kind and we also felt a confidence in their ability to care for Masood. They came and took his temperature and pulse every so often and checked that the dressing on his tummy was OK. They always spoke kindly to Masood, told him what they were going to do and why, and asked us if we were OK. The nurse who had gone to theatre to collect Masood showed us where the kitchen was, if we wanted to make tea or coffee. He also explained where the cafeteria was if we wanted to get any food and that the hospital had a prayer room, and said that if we wanted to use it, he was happy to show us where it was. They also set up a bed at Masood's bedside, so that my wife could stay with him through the night, but could still have some rest.

As Masood recovered from his operation, he was able to start having small amounts of fluids and then small amounts of food. The nurses asked us if Masood had any particular likes and dislikes before offering him any food. We liked the idea that the nurses did not make assumptions about food preferences, but asked for our advice. Also, as Masood was able to sit up, the nurse asked him if he wanted a Play Station so that he could play games.

Hakim and his grandmother, uncle and auntie came to see Masood on the day after his operation. We were a bit worried that so many people would not be able to visit at once, but the nurses just found more chairs, and even brought an additional Play Station controller, so that the boys could play games together.

Masood's recovery was unproblematic and he was ready to come home the next day. Before we brought him home, the nurse made sure that we had pain medicine and antibiotics, and that we knew how and when to give them to him. He also gave us a letter to take to our doctor and told us when we needed to go to the doctor's surgery to have the stitches removed.

We had heard a lot about the NHS before coming to Britain and now, having had first-hand experience of the service, we can see why it has such a reputation. The care that we all had was first class and we would like to thank everyone who was involved in this.

Critical Incident Analysis exercise

Using critical incident analysis, can you list all the elements from this case study that could be described as a critical incident? You may wish to refer to the work of Benner (1984) detailed in Chapter 1, but particularly think about incidents:

- in which the nurses' intervention made a difference to the care recipients;
- that were ordinary and typical;
- that captured the essence of nursing.

Commentary on the case study

The following is a list of the possible critical incidents in this case study that could be used for reflection and they have been mapped to the attributes and characteristics that service users valued in nurses as presented by Rush and Cook (2006) and Pryds-Jensen et al. (1993) as attributes of a 'caring nurse'.

Possible critical incident	Commentary	Rush and Cook (2006) and Pryds-Jensen et al. (1993) attributes and characteristics
Despite some language difficulties (understanding complex terms) the nurse made sure that the family fully understood what the doctor had told them.	It is likely that the stress and complex medical language used may have been very difficult for anyone using English as a second language and yet information giving to parents at such a critical time is essential in order to effectively care for both the parents and the child.	Competence. Communication. Knowledge of others. Demonstrates empathy. Deeply concerned and acts on the basis of ethical values and attitudes. Acts calmly to control stressful situations.
The parents were asked to sign a consent form and the nurse ensured that they fully understood what they were signing, and what was going to happen to Masood.	Consent to treatment is a very important element of care underpinned by information giving which enables 'informed' consent.	Competence. Communication.
The mother was invited to help to prepare Masood and accompany him to theatre.	The feeling of loss of control for a parent in a situation like this can be stark and matched to the child's panic and confusion over what is happening to them. By allowing the mother to care for her child and prepare him for theatre the needs of both individuals are enabled: the need of the mother to help her child, to make him better, and the need of the child for the comfort and 'normality' that his mother represents.	Competence. Compassion. Kindness. Knowledge of others. Demonstrates empathy. Timing based on intuition. Deeply concerned and acts on the basis of ethical values and attitudes. Acts calmly to control stressful situations.
When he was quite distressed (despite having had painkillers) the mother was encouraged to cuddle him and give him comfort. This helps him settle and enabled the mother to feel that she was doing something to help to alleviate her son's distress.	Again this is about trying to restore normality to the situation by enabling the mother to do what is natural in terms of comforting the child.	Compassion. Kindness. Communication. Knowledge of others. Demonstrates empathy. Timing based on intuition. Deeply concerned and acts on the basis of ethical values and attitudes. Acts calmly to control stressful situations.
They always spoke kindly to Masood, told him what they were going to do and why, and asked the parents if they were OK.	Taking time to be with care recipients, explaining what is happening, what to expect and why, and also acknowledging that it is actually alright not to feel OK are essential components of caring. It enables both honesty and the individuals to feel 'cared for': that they are important and that someone is 'there' for them.	Competence. Compassion. Kindness. Knowledge of others. Demonstrates empathy. Timing based on intuition. Generous. Honesty. Deeply concerned and acts on the basis of ethical values and attitudes. Acts calmly to control stressful situations.
They also explained where they could get drinks and food, that the hospital had a prayer room and they set up a bed so mum could stay but have some rest.	This again demonstrates how the parents are also being cared for through this process. Their nutritional and comfort needs are being addressed as are their spirituality or religious needs.	Competence. Communication. Knowledge of others. Demonstrates empathy. Love for humans. Deeply concerned and acts on the basis of ethical values and attitudes.
The nurses asked if Masood had any particular likes and dislikes before offering him any food. The nurses did not make assumptions about food preferences, but asked for advice.	All people have food preferences, but there may be particular practices associated with cultural and religious frameworks.	Competence. Knowledge of others. Practical skills.

Other possible critical incidents include the following.

- Masood knew exactly what was happening when the IV line was inserted but was kept occupied so that he did not focus on the needle going into his arm.
- The nurse told the parents to ask any questions that they had at any time, saying that if she was unable to address them, she would make sure she either found out, or got someone else to talk to them.
- On the ward, the nurses were very kind and this helped the parents to feel confidence in their ability to care for Masood.

Exercise using Gibbs' Reflective Cycle

Using Gibbs' reflective cycle (1988) (detailed in Chapter 1) to consider one of the critical incidents listed above or a different aspect of the case study, reflect further by working through each of the stages of the cycle and ensuring that you include the action you would take to improve user outcomes in the future. It may be an improved outcome for this particular user, improving care giving for future care recipients or replicating what has gone well for other care recipients.

Analysing the caring process using frameworks of knowledge

Working through a critical incident or using Gibbs' reflective cycle enables us to recognise how important it is to understand the knowledge that underpins an activity so that we can understand the way in which that knowledge is organised and applied in practice. In order to do this we will explore the physical, cognitive and emotive domains of nursing and Carper's four fundamental patterns of knowing (1978) that underpin contemporary nursing practice.

Activity

Can you think of examples of care given within this case study that fit within the
- Physical domain?
- Cognitive domain?
- Emotive domain?

Physical, cognitive and emotive domains or aspects

The physical domain

Within this case study there is little doubt that immediate and invasive (i.e. surgical) intervention is required in order to care for this child.

Therefore, the questions we need to ask about the care given are concerned with the following.

- Medical technical competence (Wilde-Larsson and Larsson, 1999) of the care givers – that is, the ability of the care giver to perform physical care in a safe and competent manner. This is demonstrated in the case study in a number of ways, such as the timely diagnosis by medical staff and the use of IV fluids and pain relief (**ESC 38**). The successful outcome of the physical care is demonstrated in Masood being discharged home the next day and experiencing an 'unproblematic' recovery.
- The physical-technical conditions (Wilde Larsson and Larsson, 1999) of the care organisation. Underlying the individual physical care of Masood is the infrastructure of the hospital, which includes having the right environment and equipment in order to facilitate care delivery (**Essence of Care Benchmark – Care Environment**). This can be as basic as having a bed to admit him to and theatre space so he can have surgery without an inappropriate wait.

Activity

List all the departments within the hospital structure that were necessary to ensure the physical-technical conditions of the organisation to enable Masood's care to be successful.

In the five attributes identified by Brilowski and Wendler (2005) in Chapter 2, which provide a good framework to consider caring, one of the attributes (actions) could relate to physical care giving. However, actions are not only about 'doing for' the care recipient but also about 'being with' them.

Nursing actions include care that:

- is physical such as inserting and caring for Masood's IV line;
- gives a feeling of 'presence' – this was demonstrated when the nurse told the parents that if she was unable to address their questions then she would make sure she either found or got someone else to talk to them, thus reassuring the parents that there were people with them at all times who could help;
- is competent – an understanding of how human and physical science interacts with the humanity of the care recipient and family is crucial to good care – this was demonstrated throughout, but one example is when the nurses recognised the need of the mother to physically prepare Masood for theatre (**ESC 10.i**); they might have been quicker or more efficient at getting children into gowns when the IV line is

attached but they recognised the need of the mother to help the child and the child to be comforted by the normality of his mother's care.

The cognitive domain

Cognitive aspects of care concern reasoning and communication (Webber, 2002) and, therefore, the way care was given to the parents in order for them to understand what was happening to their son, so that they could make decisions for him but also confront this very stressful situation with understanding. Part of this is also about information giving and receiving to attain informed consent and this will be covered in more depth below.

The Code: Standards of Conduct, Performance and Ethics for Nurses and Midwives states that nurses must:

Ensure you gain consent:

You must ensure that you gain consent before you begin any treatment or care;
You must respect and support people's rights to accept or decline treatment and care;
You must uphold people's rights to be fully involved in decisions about their care.

(NMC, 2008, p. 2)

The emotional domain

The second of Brilowski and Wendler's (2005) identified themes is 'relationship'. This case study demonstrates the ways in which the relationship built by the care-giving staff enables the trust, intimacy and responsibility shared between the child and his mother to support the care intervention. By being there for the mother and supporting her emotional need to care for her child, she is supported to be there for Masood. This is demonstrated clearly when she is encouraged to climb onto Masood's bed in theatre recovery to comfort him in his distress. The emotional support required for the child who was probably terrified by what was happening to him was most appropriately given by his mother, something even the most skilful and competent nurse could not replicate (**ESC 10.i**). This protected both the mother and the child's vulnerabilities and is a good example of 'knowing the care recipient or patient' (Tanner *et al.*, 1993), that is, having an involved rather than detached understanding of the person's situation and responses and the commitment to address vulnerability while enhancing the dignity of both.

Carper's *Fundamental Patterns of Knowing in Nursing*

Empirics

Empirics are the factual or science-based aspects of care delivery. They involve describing, explaining and predicting phenomena. Empirics can be related to the organisation of care, or the evidence on which intervention for acute appendicitis is based. Empirics would have been used by the care givers:

- to diagnose the condition and assess how quickly intervention was required;
- to decide the most effective pain relief;
- to determine the most effective surgical procedure to use;
- to prevent infection;
- for the safe use of anaesthesia.

Activity

The list above mainly concerns the empirics of 'medical' interventions.
- Can you list at least five examples of the empirics that underpin the nursing interventions in providing care for Masood and his family?

Aesthetics

The aesthetic of nursing involves not just the observation and description of a care recipient's behaviour and actions, but also an understanding of their view of what is significant in terms of needs and wants and experiences. Three of the five identified attributes that provide a good framework to consider caring, as described by Brilowski and Wendler (2005) in Chapter 2, are important here: attitude, acceptance and variability.

The attitude of a professional towards a care recipient demonstrated through their professional caring behaviours should display attributes of commitment, knowledge, skills and respect for person (Stockdale and Warelow, 2000). It enables the care recipient to feel 'cared about'. Part of this as a process is about feeling accepted, that is worthy of dignity and respect, intrinsically valuable and precious as human beings (Brilowski and Wendler, 2005). This is also about demonstrating concern about how a patient views the world, which involves active listening and responding in a way that indicates an understanding of what they are saying. In the case study this is demonstrated throughout but particularly through the continued encouragement of the mother to be involved in Masood's care and also when checking out food preferences and not making assumptions about diet based on cultural background. Core to this caring relationship is Egan's concept of unconditional acceptance: that of accepting clients as individuals entitled to respect and care but not necessarily accepting their values and behaviours which may be at odds with your own value systems (Egan, 2002) (**ESC 3.ii; 3.vi; 5.iii; 5.v**).

In order to achieve this caring relationship, variability is important because care giving is a fluid and changing skill depending on circumstances, environment and the people involved. It is also based on having respect for the identity and integrity of other human beings and being sensitive and non-judgemental. It is also about having the knowledge and skills to intervene in a way that promotes best quality of life as perceived by the patient (Russel, 2007), whatever their cultural background or their individual values or behaviours, and not imposing your own perceptions of what is best.

Activity

Think of an example of when a member of your peer group or family expressed beliefs or demonstrated behaviours that conflicted with your own value system.
- How did it make you feel?
- What was the consequence for your relationship?
- Would it be different if the person involved had been a person in your care?

Part of this sensitivity to the person's individuality is also about acknowledging their spiritual and religious beliefs and this is demonstrated in guidance from the NHS management executive:

> NHS Trusts should: make adequate provision for the spiritual needs of their patients and staff.
>
> (DH, 1992)

> NHS Staff will respect your privacy and dignity. They will be sensitive to and respect your religion, spiritual and cultural needs at all times.
>
> *Your Guide to the NHS* (DH, 2001c)

Activity

What is spirituality?
- Spend a few minutes thinking about what spirituality means to you.

We need to unpack the different meanings of spirituality if we are going to provide spiritual health care to people within a holistic context. For some people, spirituality is something that is very personal and individual while, for others, spiritual understanding is framed within a religious doctrine. The ward nurse demonstrates an important awareness of cultural differences here, without making assumptions about religious practices. Spiritual and religious understanding is important and nurses have an important role to play in assessing spiritual need and acting as a gateway to other services. Again, the ward nurse demonstrates understanding without making assumptions, by making Masood's parents aware of the availability of the prayer room (**ESC 4.1; 4.ii; 4.iii; KSF Core dimension 6 – Equality and Diversity**).

Cultural competency is important at both institutional and individual levels of health care. Cross *et al.* (1989) identify five elements that are important in the provision of culturally competent care.

Essential elements of culturally competent care:
1. Valuing diversity.
2. Having the capacity for cultural self-assessment.
3. Being conscious of the dynamics inherent when cultures interact.
4. Having institutionalised cultural knowledge.
5. Having developed adaptations of service delivery reflecting on understanding of cultural diversity.

Ethics (the moral content of nursing knowledge)

Autonomy can be defined as deliberated self-rule (Gillon, 1994) and it is therefore essential that individuals or, in the case of Masood, his parents are able to demonstrate autonomy through the process of informed consent. To proceed without gaining the informed consent of care recipients could be interpreted as physical assault against the person, or battery (Young, 1994). In order to give legally valid consent a person must have the capacity to understand and come to a decision on what is involved and to communicate that decision (Skegg, 1984). Informed consent is 'the process whereby explicit communication of information is provided and included' within the consenting process (Young, 1994) (**ESC 8.i; 8.ii**). This must include information about the risks involved.

Information giving can be complicated by the cultural background of the information giver. Meddings and Haith-Cooper (2008) in their study of cultural and language barriers in midwives recognise that a lack of commonality (due to cultural disparity) may also influence the type of information a care giver presents. An example is that if a midwife has little comprehension of a women's beliefs about childbirth, which may be very different to her own, then the information needed by that women in order to maintain her autonomy in choice cannot be achieved. A care giver must therefore endeavour to develop an understanding of the care recipient's cultural perspective of the world and, importantly, respect it as it may impact on the decision and choices made.

Activity

- Do you think that Masood's parents gave informed consent?
- What makes you draw that conclusion?
- Would the provision of an interpreter have helped?

Within this process of gaining informed consent it is also very important to consider issues of power. Practitioners need to be aware of their power in relation to the lives of their care recipient and the web of power that surrounds people who are in need of the services that practitioners can give (Brotherton and Parker, 2008). Power is 'the power to influence and control people, events or resources' (Thompson, 2003) and can be seen in positive and negative lights as demonstrated by Allen's (2000) list of different forms of power.

Forms of power:
- coercion;
- manipulation;
- domination;
- constraint;
- expertise;
- authority;
- persuasion.

Activity

- Think of examples of how Allen's forms of power (2000) might be evident in a clinical situation.
- How do you think your status as a nurse may influence the decisions made by individuals in your care?

Personal knowledge

As a human activity, based on interpersonal and therapeutic relationships, personal knowledge, gained through reflection, is fundamental to good nursing practice, as this will impact on the nature and quality of the interpersonal relationships. Care givers are able to integrate thoughts, feelings and actions by reflecting on their own practice (and its impact) in daily caring situations (Ekebergh *et al.*, 2004). Basing this on moral consciousness and meeting with the care recipient enables them to respect their life situation. It could be argued that in order to fully understand the impact of an individual's culture on their care needs it is necessary for the care giver to both understand the care recipient's culture but also to have an awareness of the impact of their own cultural norms on their care giving by developing their knowledge of self through reflection (**ESC 5.v; 9.viii**). Cultural differences could include issues about:

- personal space – some cultures are comfortable with physical closeness, seeing it as a sign of caring, while others may prefer care givers to maintain a physical distance whenever possible;
- eye contact – direct eye contact can be interpreted as aggressive or impolite and so, if an individual avoids eye contact, it may not mean that they are uninterested or shy but that they are demonstrating re-spect;
- physical contact – some cultures avoid contact with members of the opposite gender and may be very concerned with modesty and value being covered up even when being examined;
- diet – some cultures and religions prohibit certain foods and products containing food derivatives (e.g. pork-derived insulin).

(Adapted from Becze, 2007)

Activity

Think of a recent interaction with a care recipient. What impact did your cultural norms have on the:
- personal space used or maintained?
- eye contact?
- physical contact?

Interpersonal or therapeutic relationships – what is kindness?

In his letter Masood's father refers to the kindness of the care givers when expressing his satisfaction with the care experience and he is not alone in valuing kindness, as a study looking at patient satisfaction with anaesthesia demonstrates. The factor of 'kindness and regard' of the care givers was demonstrated to have the highest correlation with patient satisfaction (Capuzzo *et al.*, 2005). But what is kindness? It is based on the emotional aspect of caring, perhaps in terms of what the perceived act of kindness conjures in the emotional response of the care recipient. It seems to be about empathy (see Chapter 4) and compassion and also a level of emotional involvement and commitment from the nurse that enables the care recipients to experience closeness or a level of intimacy within this professional relationship. The attitude expressed to the care recipient based on this involvement and commitment is perceived as kindness (**ESC 5.i; 5.iii**).

The perception of kindness on one level may be the recognition and response to compassion expressed by the care giver. Compassion is a strong emotion or sentiment evoked by the recognition of another's suffering (Morse *et al.*, 1992). In her study of what patients value in nurses, Fosbinder refers to the kindness and compassion showed by nurses who go the extra mile:

> One nurse was a gem last night. She got emotional with me...she held my hand. Going by the books is good...but a gem does more ....she took a moment away from being a nurse, thinking about medicine, she was compassionate.
>
> (Fosbinder, 1994)

In our case study, in sharing the experience of the parents' suffering the expression of compassion for their suffering comforts the parents. This is strengthened by the reflexive reassurance (Morse *et al.*, 1992) given to the parents, which is a spontaneous reaction by the care giver to counteract feelings of anxiety or worry – a recognition of another's plight that evokes a response. An example of this is seen when the nurses reassure the parents that they will look after Masood while he sleeps, that explanations about what is happening are given immediately and through the constant reassurance given that, although it is not detailed in the case study, is implicit in the narrative.

Another approach to the concept of kindness may be that of its influence on the establishment of the therapeutic relationship. As an attitude towards care recipients, kindness seems to be closely related to the fostering of a therapeutic alliance and is associated with supportiveness (Sandell *et al.*, 2007).

The importance of kindness then seems to be in its role as an attitude or perceived intent to support felt by the care recipient and that therefore facilitates the care relationship. It may enable a relationship in which the care recipient perceives that the carer is there for them, is flexible, shows a keen interest and is there to help them address their problems as they arise (Escudero-Carretero *et al.*, 2007). This enables a more intimate and humane relationship leading towards participatory health care.

THE EVALUATION OF CARE

One model of quality assurance that can be adopted here is described by Donabedian (1966), who examines the evaluation of health care and describes three approaches to specifying and measuring quality – structure, process and outcome. He noted that all three are equally important in measuring the quality of care provided by a health care organisation and that they are complementary and should be used collectively to monitor quality of care.

Structure

Structure refers to human and physical resources and can include staff and policy. The structure of the organisation can be influenced by a number of factors including:

- having strong leadership at strategic (i.e. board) and operational (i.e. ward and department) level;
- adequate provision of resources such as theatre space and beds which match demand;
- having a strong organisational strategy and high-level support in the organisation (ratified at board level), which enables the organisation to achieve financial balance and national targets such as the four-hour Accident and Emergency waiting target (DH, 2004d), which Masood certainly did not breach;
- having policies in place across the organisation to ensure that issues such as infection control are dealt with, e.g., the policy of mandatory hand washing between patients with the availability of hand gels on the wards even for the family or carers to use on entering clinical areas.

Structural resources in an organisation that are of a high quality are often invisible to the care recipient as they are often the elements that underpin their experience but are not directly witnessed by them. It is more often when the structure breaks down that this is experienced directly. This would have been the case if, for example, there were no beds for Masood to go to after his surgery, or even if there had been no available theatre for a number of hours, which may have led to his appendix perforating.

Activity

From Masood's case study, do you think the structure of the health care received demonstrated a high quality? Why do you feel this?

Process

Process refers to the methods of working so may include the procedures for allocating resources or implementing clinically effective care. Ensuring clinical effectiveness is about supporting and ensuring the quality of clinical practice within the organisation, and part of this process can be the promotion of evidence-based practice. The use of clinical guidelines is one way to implement this and guidelines are based on clinical evidence, produced by clinical experts and passed through a process of rigorous checking before being ratified by the organisation. The process by which clinicians are educated about and adopt clinical guidelines is therefore part of the quality story. Process issues in the case study also include:

- good partnerships between the departments so all involved know their responsibility and Masood's journey through the different departments of the hospital is a smooth one (**ESC 13.iii; 14.iii; 17.i; 17.ii**);
- the organisation of work on the ward to which Masood was admitted;
- the process of caring for him.

Outcomes

Outcomes refer to the effect of both the structure and the process, the result of a number of individual 'outputs'. One outcome is patient satisfaction, which is very positive in the case study. This is seen in Masood's father's satisfaction that:

> I cannot fault the care that Masood received . . . and the nurse was very good, making sure that Masood knew exactly what was happening . . . (the doctor) asked our permission to give Masood some pain relief . . . The nurse made sure that we fully understood what the doctor had told us . . . [the mother] to help to prepare Masood for theatre . . . the nurses were very kind and we also felt a confidence in their ability . . .

Overall Masood's recovery was unproblematic and he was ready to go home the next day and so, in terms of the outcomes from the service provider's point of view, the episode was dealt within in a timely and evidence-based manner without complications that might have led to a longer length of stay and more financial expense, as well as the emotional and physical effect this could have had on the boy and his family.

Reflection	
Identify at least three things that you have learned from this chapter.	1. 2. 3.
How do you plan to use this knowledge within clinical practice?	1. 2. 3.
How will you evaluate the effectiveness of your plan?	1. 2. 3.
What further knowledge and evidence do you need?	1. 2. 3.

SUMMARY

- The UK is a multicultural society and the importance of culturally competent care, which recognises spiritual and cultural belief systems, is fundamental to providing good-quality, holistic care.
- It is important to recognise and acknowledge the expertise of significant others, such as parents, friends and relatives within the caring process.
- Kindness is a valued human virtue that can enable the care recipient to feel safe, valued and comforted.
- The provision of information and understanding is imperative in the provision of ethically sound care.

FURTHER READING

Dimond, B. (2004) *Legal aspects of nursing.* London: Longman
This book introduces nurses and other health care professionals to the law via everyday nursing situations of legal consequence and includes specialist chapters on paediatrics, intensive therapy units and many other areas. It takes a practical approach via fictional 'Situation' boxes that expertly highlight the relevance of the law to health care professionals' daily work.

Greenstreet, W. (ed.) (2006) *Integrating spirituality in health and social care: perspectives and practical approaches.* Oxford: Radcliffe
This book explores what is meant by spirituality and embeds it within the context of holistic care. It offers a broad view of the way that spirituality is defined and uses diagrams, exercises and case studies to aid understanding.

Meddings, F. and Haith-Cooper, M. (2008) 'Culture and communication in ethical care'. *Nursing Ethics*, 15 (1): 52–60
This article explores the ethical care of individuals from different ethnic and cultural backgrounds and the underpinning ethics of doing so.

Chapter 7

Long-term Conditions and Dignity in Care

> **The key issues that will be addressed in this chapter are:**
>
> - the importance of dignity in the provision of care;
> - supportive care at the end of life for patients and their significant others;
> - use of nursing models as tools for assessing, planning, implementing and evaluating care;
> - the importance of providing good standards of hygiene and provision of personal care;
> - the role of the nurse in providing the environment and support for a peaceful death;
> - respect for individual preferences and person-centred care.
>
> By the end of the chapter you will be able to:
> - identify critical incidents from a case study;
> - use Gibbs' reflective cycle to examine a critical incident;
> - analyse the case study using frameworks of knowledge to identify relevant issues in the care of people with long-term conditions and at the end of life;
> - use a prescribed nursing model to consider the caring process;
> - consider issues of dignity and respect for individuals in the process of care;
> - consider how the care provided in this case study could be evaluated.

INTRODUCTION

The case study in this chapter reflects the work that a nurse might undertake when working with people with long-term conditions and, in particular, supporting users and carers at the end of life. Demographic changes have led to an ageing population and an increased incidence of chronic illnesses and life-limiting conditions. While long-term conditions can affect all ages, there is an increased incidence in older age groups. This shift in the nature of disease is reflected in a number of recent policy documents. The *National Service Framework for Long Term Conditions* (DH, 2005c) focuses on neurological conditions, although the principles of management and support are applicable to all chronic conditions. The focus is on supporting people to make decisions about their care, with an emphasis on independent living where possible. However, it also acknowledges the need for palliative care services to offer both symptom relief and social, psychological, personal and spiritual care when needed.

More than half a million people aged 65 or over live in care homes (nursing and personal care) and substantial numbers end their lives in these care settings (Social Care Institute for Excellence (SCIE), 2004). There has been considerable policy attention to end-of-life care, reflecting the changing nature of disease and the need for caring and supportive services, as well as curative services in health care (DH, 2006a; *NHS End of Life Care Programme*, 2006), and the fact that increasing numbers of people are dying in care homes is also the focus of policy attention (National Council for Palliative Care, 2006). The key themes of these various policy initiatives can be summarised as:

- supporting people to support themselves where appropriate;
- supporting both service users and carers in end-of-life care decisions;
- providing holistic support to users and carers at the end of life.

In addition, there is current policy attention being focused on dignity and well-being in care: 'high quality health and social care services should be delivered in a person-centred way that respects the dignity of the individual receiving them' (DH, 2006b). This involves respecting people's right to privacy and dignity in care, listening to what people want and providing care in an appropriate environment.

THE LONG-TERM CONDITIONS AND DIGNITY IN CARE CASE STUDY

My Alfie died last year in the Beeches Nursing Home. He had a stroke nearly two years ago, shortly after our golden wedding anniversary, and the nurses in hospital felt that I would not be able to cope with looking after him at home. I wanted him to come home, but my son agreed with the nurses, and so we looked for a nursing home for him. Looking back, they were probably right, but I still wish I had been able to have him home.

The Beeches was a nice place and there were lots of different activities for the residents. I have no real complaints about the care that he received, although there were times when he could have done with a shave and it used to drive me mad when he had bits of old food in his dentures or his hair wasn't combed.

I particularly remember a red-haired nurse called Sarah. She was always cheerful, seemed to have time to spend with people and seemed to genuinely care about the residents. I always knew when she had been looking after Alfie, as he was clean-shaven, his hair was neat and tidy and his clothes were clean. One particular Sunday, I went to see Alfie as usual, and couldn't find his best shirt. Sarah was on duty, so I asked her about it. She told me that she had dressed Alfie in his best shirt, knowing that I liked him to wear it on a Sunday (I don't remember ever telling her that, but I suppose I might have done). Some of his morning tea had got spilt on the shirt and Alfie had got quite agitated, rubbing at the dirty patch and trying to communicate although, of course, he couldn't talk. Sarah had taken the shirt and sponged out the stain and was just waiting for it to dry. I think she got into trouble from the Matron, because it is not really part of the nurse's job to do that, but I hope not. That gesture of kindness meant such a lot to me and I know it would have done to Alfie as well. He always took such pride in his appearance and in being respectable, however tough things were.

Sarah was on duty when Alfie died. I had been telephoned the night before and told that he had had a further stroke and that he was gravely ill. My son Neil was on holiday with the family in Gran Canaria, so I got a taxi straight to the Beeches. My Alfie was unconscious, but he looked surprisingly peaceful and I noticed that his hair had been combed and he had clean pyjamas and bed linen. This might not seem important to some people, but it meant such a lot to me. I felt that Alfie looked really cared for and it seemed to me that that indicated that the nurses cared about him, and were not just going through the motions.

I was sitting with Alfie, holding his hand, when Sarah came in that morning. She asked me if I wanted her to sit with me. I explained that I had rung Neil and he was on his way back from Gran Canaria, but I would be grateful if she could spare the time to sit with me. She explained that even though it seemed that Alfie might be deeply unconscious, we couldn't be sure that he couldn't hear us and that if I wanted to talk to him, that would be OK, and might help him to feel my presence. She sat with me for a while, often in silence, until she had to go and do something else. I did talk to Alfie and told him how much I loved him, and reminisced about some of the wonderful things that we had done together throughout our lives. Looking back on it now, I am glad that I did this – it felt as though I said goodbye properly to Alfie and I like to think that it gave him some comfort in his final hours.

Unfortunately, Alfie died before Neil could get back from Gran Canaria. Again, Sarah came and sat with me. I have never felt comfortable crying in front of other people, but couldn't help it, and Sarah was amazingly kind. I don't remember her saying much, but it felt quite natural when she put her arm around me on one occasion or another time when she placed her hand over mine, I felt comforted. I talked to her a lot about my life with Alfie and she sat and listened. I never felt that she was impatient to get on with other things or that she didn't have the time to sit with me. We seemed to sit together for a long time before my sister arrived, although I can't be sure exactly how long it was.

I still miss Alfie dreadfully, but I am able to look back fondly on my many happy memories of our life together. I feel comforted that he had a peaceful death and that he was so well cared for in the hours leading up to his death. I shall never forget the nurses at The Beeches and, in particular, Sarah's kindness and thoughtfulness. When I thanked her, she seemed almost embarrassed and said that she was just doing her job, but it was so much more to me.

Critical incident analysis exercise

Using critical incident analysis, as described at the end of Chapter 1, can you list all the elements from this case study that could be described as a critical incident? Include examples of practice that are either good or bad as well as incidents that can give insight into practice, focusing specifically on why it was successful or could have been improved in some way. Give at least three positive examples and an example where the nurse could have improved the outcome for the service user.

Commentary on the case study

On page 118 is a list of the possible critical incidents that could be used for reflection on this case study. These have been mapped to the attributes and characteristics that service users valued in nurses as presented by Rush and Cook (2006) and Pryds-Jensen *et al.*'s (1993) attributes of a 'caring nurse'.

Exercise using Gibbs' Reflective Cycle

Use Gibbs' reflective learning cycle (see Chapter 1) to reflect on one of the critical incidents that you have identified. Work through the stages of the cycle, ensuring you include the actions that you would take to improve user outcomes in the future. This may relate to improving the outcomes for this particular care recipient, or replicating positive actions in this scenario for other care recipients.

Analysing the caring process using frameworks of knowledge

Working through a critical incident or using Gibbs' reflective cycle enables us to recognise how important it is to understand the knowledge

Possible critical incident	Commentary	Rush and Cook (2006) and Pryds-Jensen *et al.* (1993) attributes and characteristics
Alfie's discharge from hospital.	This involves difficult decisions by a number of people, balancing different viewpoints and wishes with the needs of the care recipient.	Communication.
Alfie was always well groomed and his dentures were cleaned when Sarah was on duty.	This was important, as it demonstrates that Sarah was using her nursing knowledge in a person-centred way to address Alfie's functional needs.	Practical skills. Competence. Knowledge of others.
Sarah recognised why Alfie got agitated after spilling his tea.	This demonstrates intuitive knowledge, as Sarah was able to recognise what Alfie was trying to communicate and responded in an appropriate way to reduce the agitation.	Knowledge of others. Knowledge. Compassion. Kindness.
Alfie looked peaceful and had clean sheets and pyjamas.	This action demonstrates a commitment from the care staff and an understanding of the importance of comfort.	Compassion. Love for humans.
Sarah told Alfie's wife that she could still talk to him even though he was deeply unconscious.	This demonstrates an empathic understanding, where Sarah uses her knowledge to empower Alfie's wife, so that she feels that she is doing something important and feels less helpless.	Knowledge. Compassion.
Sarah sat unhurriedly with Alfie's wife until her sister arrived.	This demonstrates a compassion for Alfie's wife and an empathic understanding.	Demonstrate empathy. Timing based on intuition. Kindness. Communication. Compassion.

that underpins an activity so that we can understand the way in which that knowledge is organised and applied in practice. In order to do this we will explore the physical, cognitive and emotive domains of nursing and Carper's four fundamental patterns of knowing that underpin contemporary nursing practice.

Physical, cognitive and emotive domains or aspects

Activity

Can you think of examples of care given within this case study that fit within the:
- Physical domain?
- Cognitive domain?
- Emotive domain?

The physical domain

There are a lot of elements of physical care that Alfie requires during his entire stay in the nursing home and during the period of critical illness prior to his death. Within this case study, Alfie's wife stresses the importance of oral hygiene and personal cleanliness, which we can see fits in with Roper *et al.*'s model of activities of daily living (2000), and is a fundamental human need (Maslow, 1962). In addition, there is physical care of the dying person, involving comfort needs, such as the provision of a comfortable and clean environment (**KSF Core dimension 3 – Health, Safety and Security; Essence of Care Benchmark – Care Environment**), as well as some physical needs that are not directly discussed in this case study, such as relief or management of pain, hydration and other symptom control (see Goff, in Heath and Schofield, 1999, for a detailed discussion of nursing older people at the end of life).

Physical care is important, but so is the manner in which it is carried out. In providing physical care, nurses may be involved in the use of physical touch in areas of the body that would not normally be touched within a social relationship.

> The work of nurses is about caring for bodies. This is a problem in that they must attend to those bodily functions, which have, in a 'civilised' society, become taboo.
>
> (Nettleton, 2006, p. 124)

Lawler (1991) argues that nurses therefore must find strategies to negotiate this invasion of privacy with care recipients, so that the care recipient feels safe and that they are not violated by the physical touch. Emotional intimacy is also important here. Ersser (1998) argues that a close relationship between nurse and care recipient provides opportunities for the expression of anxieties and this can ease the embarrassment and discomfort that people may feel when intimate physical care is being provided. Thus good physical care is not just about the technical or physical task, but involves the humanistic elements of an interpersonal relationship.

The cognitive domain

The case study demonstrates the nurse's commitment to the holistic care of individuals and the value that is placed on the total care and well-being of individuals. For example, Alfie's wife comments on the fact that there were always plenty of activities for the residents to become involved in. In addition, Sarah's willingness to sit with Alfie's wife demonstrates the value that she attached to the care of both the service user and their carer.

The emotional domain

> **Activity**
>
> Before reading the next section, go back to the case study and highlight all the elements of care that could fall into the emotional domain.

There are a number of emotional aspects of care demonstrated in this case study. The indirect communication and the small but important gestures of touch that Sarah uses indicate an emotional attachment and context to the care that Sarah provides for Alfie's wife (McCorkle, 1974; Chang, 2001). In addition, Alfie's wife remembers Sarah sitting with her, but not saying very much. This demonstrates Benner's (1984) notion of presencing, where verbal communication and touch are not the only means of communicating emotional support. Being with someone and sharing a mutual space and situation can form an emotional connection. In addition, sitting with someone without necessarily feeling the need to speak or physically comfort demonstrates respect for the individual's own way of coping, allowing them time for personal reflection.

Carper's *Fundamental Patterns of Knowing in nursing*

This case study allows us to explore the different dimensions of nursing knowledge as detailed by Carper (1978).

Empirics

The empirical knowledge demonstrated in this case study is in respect of the fundamental care that Alfie experienced during his entire stay in the nursing home. Nurses will have used factual knowledge to provide evidence-based oral and personal hygiene care (**Essence of Care Benchmark – Personal and Oral Hygiene; ESC 2.vi**) (Geissler and McCord, 1986; Griffiths and Boyle, 2005; Duffin, 2008). In addition, Sarah uses factual knowledge about unconscious people's ability to hear in her advice to Alfie's wife. There is also some evidence of factual knowledge about what constitutes a good death here and the ways in which the nurse can facilitate this. The importance of saying goodbye to someone is acknowledged, which is an important component of acceptance of the impending death (Kubler-Ross, 1970) and the preparedness for the loss (Kellehear, 1990).

The concept of the 'good death':
• awareness of dying;
• adjustments and preparations for death;

- relinquishing of roles;
- responsibilities and duties;
- making of farewells with others.

(Kellehear, 1990)

Aesthetics

The art of nursing emphasises the qualitative aspects of nursing practice, which may be practised in conjunction with the scientific (empirical) aspects of nursing (Peplau, 1952). However, Peplau goes further in stating that, at times, people are 'touched (literally and figuratively) and sometimes changed at a very personal level by the art nurses practice' (1988, p. 9). This can be seen clearly in this case study, where Alfie's wife states that 'I shall never forget the nurses at The Beeches and, in particular, Sarah's kindness and thoughtfulness'.

These elements of nursing are difficult to quantify, but clearly have an enormous impact on care recipients and carers, as evidenced by the following statement by Alfie's wife: 'When I thanked her, she seemed almost embarrassed and said that she was just doing her job, but it was so much more to me'.

In addition, Sarah demonstrates intuitive knowledge in her understanding of Alfie's distress and her attention to detail in ensuring that his best shirt was clean for him to wear on the Sunday. We have no way of knowing whether or not Alfie's wife had mentioned anything about Alfie wearing his best shirt on Sundays, but what is important here is that Sarah used creative thinking to establish the source of Alfie's distress and to provide care that demonstrated a deep-rooted subjective understanding of the particular issues (Chinn and Kramer, 1995). This intuitive knowledge is also demonstrated in Sarah's presencing and empathic understanding when she sits with Alfie's wife following his death.

Ethical knowledge

While there are ethical dilemmas that people may face at the end of life (Turner, 1997; Blank and Merrick, 2005), Carper's concept of ethical knowledge in nursing also relates to the moral decision-making at an individual level. Within this case study, Sarah makes a decision to spend time sitting with Alfie's wife, and the experience for Alfie's wife is that this was unhurried and she did not have the sense that Sarah needed to rush off and do anything else. It would be naïve to assume that there were no other nursing activities that Sarah could have been involved in, but she made a moral decision to prioritise the emotional support of Alfie's wife until her sister arrived and was able to offer her support. These decisions are difficult to make and reflect complex processes of priority setting and negotiation (**ESC 16.ii; 16.iii; 16.v**).

Personal knowledge

Sarah demonstrates a great deal of personal knowledge in this case study, although there are times when she seems not to fully appreciate the impact of her personal input and approach to Alfie's care ('When I thanked her, she seemed almost embarrassed, and said that she was just doing her job'). Again, we have no way of knowing what Sarah's personal experiences were, or how long she had been nursing, but we can see how her personal characteristics impact on the care that Alfie and his wife received, in her attention to detail and subjective understanding of the situation. She also seems to be comfortable with the silences as she sits with Alfie's wife, demonstrating a critical awareness of self and the therapeutic relationship and a genuineness that leads to trust and companionship between the two women.

Activity

- What knowledge of self does Sarah demonstrate in this case study?
- How does this relate to Davies and O'Berle's (1990) six elements of care: valuing; connecting; empowering; finding meaning; doing for; preserving integrity (see Chapter 4)?

We can see from this case study that the process of caring is complex and involves knowledge in a number of different dimensions. Watson (1985) provides a theory of nursing that seeks to balance the scientific and humanistic aspects of nursing, where she emphasises the interpersonal nature of nursing and the inter-relationship between empirics and aesthetics through the humanistic elements of caring that satisfy human needs.

> A person's mind and emotions are windows to the soul. Nursing care can be and is physical, procedural, objective, and factual, but at the highest level of nursing the nurses' human care responses, the human care transactions and the nurses' presence in the relationship transcend the physical and material world...and make contact with the person's emotional and subjective world as the route to the inner self.
>
> (Watson, 1985, p. 50)

> **Activity**
>
> Factors integral to the caring process:
> - cultivation of sensitivity to self and others;
> - development of a helping-trusting relationship;
> - promotion of acceptance of positive and negative feelings;
> - provision for a supportive, protective and corrective mental, physical, socio-cultural and spiritual environment;
> - assistance with the human needs of gratification.
>
> (Watson, 1985, pp. 9--10)
>
> Identify ways in which these elements of caring are demonstrated in the case study.

Watson's theory is useful for analysing the positive elements of care that Alfie and his wife received. Within her humanistic philosophy, she emphasises the role of self within the therapeutic relationship and that self-reflection leads to a genuineness and authenticity in the nurse that enables her/him to self-actualise and foster growth and potential in those that they come into contact with. Thus, the self-reflection on one's own feelings can lead to a sensitivity not only to one's own emotions, but also to the others that the nurse interacts with, enabling a more genuine person-to-person interaction. This can be seen in the way that Sarah approaches Alfie's wife, both before his impending death and after his death. The appropriate use of touch and demonstration of emotional support when she puts her arm around Alfie's wife demonstrates a sensitivity to both self and others. She demonstrates that she is comfortable with this form of intimate contact and she uses it in an appropriate manner to offer sensitive support to Alfie's wife. Sarah also shows sensitivity in the way that she informs Alfie's wife that it is appropriate to talk to Alfie, while Alfie's wife's response demonstrates that a trusting/helping relationship has developed.

Watson (1985) further emphasises the importance of environmental context for a caring and trusting relationship to exist. Comfort, safety and protection are important here and from the case study we can identify the importance for Alfie's wife of the fact that he was in clean pyjamas, had clean bed linen and had had his hair combed. These are more than physical elements of caring, in that they demonstrate a positive regard for the individuals. The environment where Alfie's wife has the space to be with Alfie, without interruptions, is also important. Sarah also demonstrates a degree of skill here, in providing a safe environment for Alfie's wife to express vulnerabilities.

In his theory of malignant social psychology, Kitwood (1997) explores ways that communication and environment can contribute to the negative experiences of people who have dementia. While this theory is related specifically to the care of people with dementia, the principles can be applied elsewhere, reinforcing the principle that positive regard and the facilitation of human growth and potential is multifaceted and requires consideration of factors other than the task of providing care. Positive regard for individuals can be fostered through the provision of a safe environment for the expression of vulnerabilities (Kitwood, 1997). Watson (1985) argues that nurses often work with people as they are facing stressful or threatening situations, and part of the carative focus of nursing involves providing comfort, safety and privacy so that people can face those vulnerabilities in a way that is comfortable. Thus, Sarah not only provides a physical environment that is comfortable, safe and private, but also demonstrates positive regard for Alfie's wife through the implicit communication that she has as much time as needed, as well as through her willingness to listen (**KSF Core dimension – Health, Safety and Security; Essence of Care Benchmark – Care Environment**).

Caring is therefore a complex process that involves the interplay of empirical, aesthetic, ethical and personal knowledge. So how can nurses provide holistic care, offering appropriate support and intervention in a person-centred way?

NURSING MODELS

The use of nursing models offers one way of organising complexities of care. Nursing models provide a way of conceptualising a situation and making the different elements of a complex situation explicit. In addition, the model demonstrates the relationship between these different elements and helps us to conceptualise the holistic nature of the situation (Kershaw and Salvage, 1986). Nursing models give a framework for the application of the different stages of the nursing process. Thus, within the case study, Alfie's hygiene needs are assessed by Sarah, appropriate care is planned and then evaluated on an ongoing basis. The outcome can be evaluated not only in terms of the maintenance of his personal hygiene, but also in terms of the dignity and self-esteem for both Alfie and his wife.

Therefore models provide us with tools to help to identify and assess needs, explore solutions to problems, implement and evaluate care (**ESC 9.i**). There are a number of different models that look at holistic nursing practice from different theoretical perspectives. When using these models, we may select elements of them that are relevant to the individual we are providing care for, so that that care can be individualised and appropriate. For the purpose of analysing Alfie's care, Roper *et al.*'s (2000) model of activities of daily living has been selected, partly because it is widely used in practice, and therefore may be more familiar to the reader, and partly because it offers a tool for the assessment, planning, implementation and evaluation of nursing care in process context (Roper *et al.*, 2000).

Within this model, Roper *et al.* identify 12 activities of living, and nursing is viewed as the activities that may help people 'to prevent, alleviate, solve or cope with problems' (Roper *et al.*, 2000) related to these activities of living. The 12 activities of daily living are:

- maintaining a safe environment;
- communicating;
- breathing;
- eating and drinking;
- eliminating;
- personal cleansing and dressing;
- controlling body temperature;
- mobilising;
- working and playing;
- expressing sexuality;
- sleeping;
- dying.

Problems may be actual or potential and activities may be influenced by physical, psychological, socio-cultural, environmental and politico-economic factors (Roper *et al.*, 2000). The model is concerned with understanding the person's place on the dependence/independence spectrum and how nursing interventions can provide individualised care within this context.

Activity

Using the information provided in the case study, identify the most relevant activities of daily living that the nurse would focus on when caring for Alfie.

The most obvious activities that are mentioned in this case study are: personal cleansing and dressing; working and playing; and dying. However, it must be borne in mind that, in providing holistic care to someone with long-term care needs at the dependency end of the spectrum of activity, the nurse would need to assess, plan, implement and evaluate care in all 12 activities of living.

Working and playing are important aspects of care for older people, as purposeful and meaningful activity not only enhances quality of life and demonstrates respect for individuals, but may also contribute therapeutic benefits. A number of studies have shown that purposeful activity in older age has health benefits in terms of physical health (McMurdo, 2000), mental health (Audit Commission, 2002) and general well-being and self-esteem (McClymont, 1999). Alfie's wife evaluates the care home positively because 'there were lots of different activities for the residents'. This demonstrates the potential for purposeful activity for residents as well as a focus on individualised care, where residents have a range of activities that they can choose from.

While dying might seem at first glance to be strange as an activity of daily living, helping people to die in comfort and supporting their carers is a fundamental aspect of care across the lifespan and was embodied in the cradle-to-grave philosophy of universal access to health care on the inception of the National Health Service in 1948. More recently the *National Health Services End of Life Care* guidelines have stressed that:

> End of life care requires an active compassionate approach that treats, comforts and supports individuals who are living with or dying from progressive or chronic life threatening conditions.

> Such care is sensitive to personal, cultural and spiritual values, beliefs and practices and encompasses support for families and friends up to and including the period of bereavement.
> (Ross, Fisher *et al.*, 2000, p. 9,
> cited in *NHS End of Life Care Programme*, 2006)

An important aspect of care of the dying and their families and friends is the concept of dignity and respect. In December 2007, the *Daily Telegraph* newspaper reported on a coroner's narrative verdict following the death of an 85-year-old man in a care home earlier that year. The Coroner stated that the man was:

> treated like a parcel in the last few weeks of his life with insufficient emphasis placed on his wellbeing and care . . .I can only hope that [. . .] was so withdrawn in his last few days at the home that he was not aware of the appalling care he was receiving.
> (*Daily Telegraph*, 15 December 2007)

To be treated with dignity and respect is a fundamental human right and is enshrined in the Human Rights Act 1998. In November 2006 Ivan Lewis (MP), the Minister for Care Services, launched 'The Dignity in Care Campaign' in health and social care services (**ESC 3.iii; 3.iv**). Although it has been acknowledged that there have been significant improvements in older people's access to services, concerns remain that this is at the expense of dignity and respect for individual care requirements and privacy. The Social Care Institute for Excellence (SCIE) (2006) has identified the following ten challenges for dignity in care:

- zero tolerance for all forms of abuse;
- support people with the same respect you would want for yourself or a member of your family;
- treat each person as an individual by offering a personalised service;
- enable people to maintain the maximum possible level of independence, choice and control;
- listen and support people to express their needs and wants;
- respect people's right to privacy;
- ensure people feel able to complain without fear of retribution;
- engage with family members and carers as care partners;
- assist people to maintain confidence and a positive self-esteem;
- act to alleviate people's loneliness and isolation.

(ESC 3.v; 3.vi)

Activity

In what ways did the care home promote dignity in care for Alfie?

Sturdy (2008) argues that nurses are in a position of privilege in the caregiving relationship, in that they engage with people at a time when they are at their most vulnerable. An evaluation by the Healthcare Commission in 2007 identified the following areas where older people were most often treated with indignity in health care environments:

- patients were addressed in an inappropriate manner or spoken about as if they were not there;
- people were not given information or did not have their consent sought or wishes considered;
- people were left in soiled clothes or exposed in an embarrassing manner;
- appropriate food or help with eating was not given;
- people were placed in mixed-sex accommodation.

Nurses have a duty to ensure that people are protected and treated with respect when they enter the alien environments of health care provision. The attention to Alfie's hygiene needs and personal grooming demonstrates a respect for him as an individual, and an engagement at a subjective level that understands the importance of basic care to the sense of personal integrity and well-being for both Alfie and his wife. In this sense, we can see that the care staff (and Sarah in particular) demonstrated a respect for the care recipient and carer.

Furthermore, both Alfie and his wife are respected and treated with dignity during the dying process. Sudnow (1976) argued that the concept of death in contemporary society has become increasingly ambiguous and difficult to define due to technological developments in health care and longer dying trajectories. He identified three definitions of death.

1. Biological death – the cessation of heart and respiratory activity.
2. Clinical death – the cessation of brain activity.
3. Social death – this is where the individual is treated as though they have died before the actual point of biological death has been reached. He gives the example of nurses packing up some of the belongings of an individual in preparation for their impending death.

Again, we can see that Alfie and his wife were treated with respect and dignity up until the point of death and in the immediate period of bereavement. Rather than treating Alfie as socially dead, Sarah, through her suggestion that Alfie's wife continue to talk to him, showed respect for Alfie as a person and for his relationship with his wife. She also showed respect for Alfie's wife through her verbal and non-verbal communications as she sat with her following Alfie's death and demonstrated a willingness to be with her and to listen when she wished to talk about Alfie.

THE EVALUATION OF CARE

The discussion so far has identified a number of theoretical frameworks for identifying and analysing elements of the caring process in this case study. But how can the care be evaluated? One way to consider the success of this care episode is to use Huycke and All's (2000) evaluative framework, which considers outcomes of care from the perspective of providers, payers, public and patients.

Providers

Providers (in this case, the nursing home) would be interested in the process and outcomes of care, which include staff having the knowledge to deliver appropriate care and the fact that the required patient outcomes were achieved. It seems clear that the nursing staff in general provided a high quality of care in this nursing home, although there are some areas where improvements could be made.

In this case study, questions might be asked about the quality measurement tools that are used within the care home to ensure continuing good standards. Questions might also be asked about how elements of good practice are identified and disseminated in keeping with the *Dignity in Care* agenda (DH, 2006b).

Payers

Payers are the general public in terms of taxpayers or private contributors, who might be interested in the value for money achieved through the interventions undertaken and the quality of the care provided. For example, Sarah's interventions here may have helped Alfie's wife to manage her grief. Seale (1998, p. 193) defines grief as the 'reaction to extreme damage to the social bond'. It seems evident from this case study that Alfie and his wife have a caring relationship that has endured for over 50 years and, therefore, there is the potential for great loss with the fracturing of the social bond. However, the fact that Alfie's dignity and identity were maintained right until the end of his life are important as his wife remembers his integrity as a person. Bradbury (1998) has argued that in the grief process, people go through a process of discourse, identifying whether the death was a good or bad death. A bad death can lead to complicated grief and may be associated with spoiled identity, a lack of preparedness for the death and a lack of opportunity to say goodbye (Littlewood, 1992; Riches and Dawson, 2001). While it would be too simplistic to assume that Alfie's wife would not have a complicated grieving process, the fact that she states that she felt comforted that he had a peaceful death is important. It may be that the quality of care that she received helped in her grief resolution and thus prevented a need for treatment, which would have involved additional costs to taxpayers.

Public

Public bodies, such as the Commission for Social Care Inspection (CSCI) are responsible for evaluating quality of care in nursing homes and would therefore be concerned with the care and treatment of residents. Questions that might be asked:

- Are all residents treated with respect and dignity?
- Is the privacy of residents respected?
- Are carers involved as care partners?

Again, from this case study, we can see that there are many elements of good practice. Although Alfie's wife is clearly engaged with providing comfort to him in his final hours, we might wish to ask further questions about the degree of involvement that carers have in developing activities and in the care process.

Patients

In this case study, we would evaluate the care from Alfie's wife's perspective.

Activity

- How might Alfie's wife have evaluated the care he received?
- What evidence can you find in the case study and the preceding discussion that has led you to this conclusion?

Reflection	
Identify at least three things that you have learned from this chapter.	1. 2. 3.
How do you plan to use this knowledge within clinical practice?	1. 2. 3.
How will you evaluate the effectiveness of your plan?	1. 2. 3.
What further knowledge and evidence do you need?	1. 2. 3.

SUMMARY
- Good quality of care takes account of people's privacy and dignity and provides a safe environment for people to express their vulnerabilities.

- Palliative care is an important part of contemporary nursing care and involves care for both the dying person and their significant others. Good quality of care that treats the dying person with respect and dignity can ameliorate the bereavement process.
- Nursing models help to provide a framework to enable the nursing process and provide person-centred care that respects individual needs and preferences.

FURTHER READING

Department of Health (2006b) *The Dignity in Care Campaign*. London: HMSO.
Not only does this set out the agenda for dignity in care, but it also provides useful guidance and examples of positive practice.

Costello, J. (2004) *Nursing the dying patient: caring in different contexts*. Basingstoke: Palgrave Macmillan
This is an accessible book that explores end-of-life care in a variety of health care contexts, and discusses the importance of context on the way that care is provided. Case studies are used to illustrate the discussion.

Payne, S., Seymour, J. and Ingleton, C. (2004) *Palliative care nursing: principles and evidence for practice*. Maidenhead: McGraw-Hill
This book provides a comprehensive discussion of concepts relevant to end-of-life care, and explores the evidence base and policy context for practices at the end of life.

Roper, N. (1988) *Principles of nursing in process context* (4th ed.). London: Churchill Livingstone
This book guides the reader through the 12 activities of daily living, using the nursing process as a framework to guide practice. Although some of the evidence base is now dated, this still provides a useful starting point for an understanding of holistic care.

Tanner, D. and Harris, J. (2008) *Working with older people*. London: Routledge in association with Community Care
Although this is primarily aimed at social work students, this book provides some important debates about the nature of ageing and provision of care and support for older people and their carers, which are relevant to nursing practice. It uses activities to engage the learner and encourage critical reflection.

Chapter 8

Nursing in the Twenty-first Century

The key issues that will be addressed in this chapter are:

- the dominance of the biomedical model of health care and the impact on nursing developments;
- the management of UK health care in the late twentieth and early twenty-first century and the emphasis on efficiency and cost containment;
- the challenges of providing care within twenty-first century health care;
- the future challenges to nursing and the role of nurse education.

By the end of this chapter, you should be able to:

- understand the relevance of the political and economic context for caring in the twenty-first century;
- consider the impact of a target-led NHS on caring imperatives;
- discuss the impact on nursing of working within a biomedical framework of health care provision;
- describe the current policy challenges to the focus on 'cure';
- understand the concept of 'emancipatory' nursing.

THE CONTEXT OF CARE

Throughout the twentieth century and into the twenty-first century, nursing care has grown up in a system of health care dominated by a scientific model of medical care, with the emphasis on cure. As argued in Chapter 1, this biomedical framework has increasingly replaced religious and informal health care as the dominant mode of health care organisation. Turner (1995) argues that within this health care organisation, nurses have been subject to a dual line of authority. On the one hand, they are subject to the rules and regulations of a bureaucratic system of health care organisation while, at the same time, they are subject to the medical authority that is assumed because of the dominance of the curative system of health care. Peacock and Nolan (2000) argue that this has been particularly apparent since the inception of the National Health

Service in 1948, which has been described as an 'illness-obsessed service, interested only in disability, disease and death' (Annual Report of the Chief Medical Officer, 1973, cited by Peacock and Nolan, 2000, pp. 1066–7) – it is, in fact, a 'National Illness Service'.

Activity

Consider the consequences of this environment for the pursuit of care and holistic practice.

Nettleton (2006) identifies the following imperatives of a biomedical model of health care.

- The mechanistic nature of care – the analogy of car maintenance is often used here. In the same way as the car is made up of a number of different components, the body can be broken down into its component parts and each part can be treated independently.
- Mind–body dualism – this is where the mind and body are seen as separate entities, not influencing one another, and it is associated with the work of the nineteenth-century philosopher, Descartes. Since the body was seen as a physical entity, it could be separated from the metaphysical entity of the mind (Moon and Gillespie, 1995).
- Reductionism – the biomedical model is reductionist, in that it separates the physical body from social and psychological and environmental processes, with the emphasis on curing the physical malfunction, caused through trauma, germs or genetics.

Activity

- Thinking about the case study in Chapter 3, how would George have been treated using a purely biomedical model?
- How effective would it have been?

- The doctrine of specific aetiology – this emerged from the germ theory of the nineteenth century, where specific causal agents could be identified for the different infectious diseases, which were the major causes of mortality and morbidity at the time. Thus, if a specific cause could be found, a specific treatment could be identified that would 'fix the problem'. The human context was therefore ignored or secondary to the specific 'fix'.
- Cure became focused on technology, whether in terms of pharmacological interventions or in terms of invasive surgical procedures.

In 2005/06, medicines accounted for 10 per cent of NHS expenditure, with a total cost of £10.3 billion.

The cost of prescribing in primary care has increased at an average of 7.5 per cent per year in the past 10 years, and at an even faster rate in secondary care.

(NHS Information Centre, 2007)

Nettleton (2006) further argues that medicine came to be seen as the only valid and objective way of understanding health and health care, and therefore became the dominant perspective in the developing health care system of the nineteenth and twentieth centuries. This has had implications for nursing, as it emerged as an occupation within the context of this dominance of the scientific paradigm, with the emphasis on technical efficiency and little emphasis on 'caring'.

Activity

- Looking at the case study in Chapter 6, how different would Masood's father's letter be if the care he had received was purely about the surgical intervention and his parents' needs and involvement had been ignored?
- If this had been the case, do you think his physical recovery would have been so speedy?

The focus on instrumental care

Since the 1960s, nursing theorists from various theoretical standpoints have re-emphasised the importance of caring, distinguishing between the science and art of care. The science of care is that care that can be empirically measured, while the art of care involves humanistic and more qualitative aspects of care.

Science of care	Art of care
Aims at universals	Quality
Quantification	Freedom
Replicability	Style

Pepin (1992) identified two types of caring: instrumental caring and affective caring. Instrumental care involves scientific nursing actions, as discussed throughout the previous chapters in relation to Carper's (1978) patterns of scientific knowing in nursing. Affective caring is concerned with humanistic aspects of care, focusing on the art of nursing, as defined by Carper (1978) and discussed in relation to various theorists' work throughout this book.

Various writers have argued that the scientific revolution and the emphasis on technical methods of treatment and diagnosis have led to an emphasis on instrumental care, at the expense of affective care (Peacock and Nolan, 2000; Jossens and Ganley, 2006). However, it also has to be acknowledged that instrumental care is important in the delivery of holistic care and technical competence is an important element of caring. As Fry (1991) states, other elements of caring will lose their potency if the nurse is not competent. Morrison (1991) reinforces this, arguing that there is a mismatch between nurses' and patients' perceptions of important aspects of care. From his repertory grid study, he concluded that physical care is more important to patients, but psychosocial care is emphasised more by nurses. It could therefore be argued that patients value affective care only when good physical care is present.

Despite theoretical claims that nurses have reasserted the importance of affective care (Sourial, 1997), research also suggests that nurses themselves value instrumental care, and this is associated with the status and value of technical medical care. In a longitudinal qualitative study, Randle (2001) found that nurses constructed their self-esteem by engagement in the more technical aspects of care, which they saw as having higher worth and status because of their association with the skills and knowledge base of medicine. While they might also value the humanistic elements of care, time constraints led to a need to prioritise, and this led to an increased focus on the technical components of care.

This focus on technical care has been further expanded because of the political, economic and bureaucratic climate within which health care is delivered (Jossens and Ganley, 2006). In one sense, medical science has been a victim of its own success, in that people are now living longer, infant mortality in the Western world has dramatically decreased and there are general improvements in the quality of life, although inequalities persist (Acheson Report, DH 1998). In addition, people's expectations of health care have risen, with increased availability of information (Hardey, 1999).

These demographic imperatives and changing expectations have led to increased demands on health care (Allsop, 1984), with implications for resources in terms of both time and cost. This is further complicated by the efficiency drive in health care and the need for quicker throughputs in the health care system. Thus there is increased pressure on clinical staff to reach targets and ensure that people have access to care within appropriate timescales. The implications of this are that aspects of caring that are more difficult to measure may be sacrificed in the pursuit of efficiency and achievement of targets. A Royal College of Nursing Employment Survey found that 55 per cent of nurses stated that they were too busy to provide the right quality of care (Ball and Pike, 2005).

> Time constraints require healing care to be replaced by techno-logical imperatives for rapid and early hospital discharge.
>
> (Jossens and Ganley, 2006, p. 17)

An example of this was seen in the case study where the nurse on the dermatology ward was too busy to find the care recipient a jug to urinate into, using the excuse that she was not her named nurse.

Caring in a resource-challenged health service

Trying to care in a context of economic rationalism can be difficult for both the carer and cared for (Warelow, 1996). At present, nursing care is shaped by the social structures of the institutions of care, lower staffing profiles, higher nursing workloads and increased technology. So, within a finance- and time-constrained environment, how can capacity to 'care' be identi-fied? Health care provision is a political and economic activity, and nursing care operates within these parameters. Since the inception of the NHS, there have been concerns about the rising cost of health care (Klein, 1995), but this has been of particular concern since the 1980s, with the need to cut public expenditure to manage inflation (Ham, 1999). With budgets for health care growing more slowly than had been anticipated in the 1980s and early 1990s, the focus in health care became concerned with improv-ing efficiency of services while at the same time containing the costs.

> The health care system that is supposedly responsible for caring for people is highly bureaucratised with dominating structures that increasingly are driven by efficiency, profit and productivity.
>
> (Chooporian, 1986, p. 48)

Although the Conservative governments of the 1980s and 1990s imple-mented the efficiency reforms, they have continued under the New Labour government, which was elected in 1997 and has invested signifi-cantly in the NHS, but that financial investment has been predicated on reform. In the White Paper, *The New NHS: Modern, Dependable*, the government set out six principles to guide reforms in the health service:

- renew the NHS as a genuinely national service;
- make the delivery of health care against these national standards a matter of local responsibility;
- get the NHS to work in partnership;
- improve efficiency so that every pound in the NHS is spent to

maximise the care for patients;
- shift the focus on to quality of care, so that excellence is guaranteed to all patients;
- rebuild public confidence in the NHS.

(DH, 1997)

Target-setting

The monitoring of performance and efficiency is an important part of the management of health care and setting of targets has been a major management tool within this modernisation strategy in health care. Target-setting helps to measure performance and increase the accountability of the service. Targets need to be related to actions that are effective, achievable and can be monitored through indicators.

Targets are set, for example, for patients to be seen in Accident and Emergency departments (see Chapter 4), there is pressure on in-patient beds, requiring quicker discharge of patients and social services departments are fined if community care arrangements cannot be met when a person has been deemed to be medically fit for discharge (Community Care Act, 2003). These standards are also emphasised through various National Service Frameworks and plans relating to different disease areas such as cancer, and shorter waiting times.

The NHS Cancer Plan set new cancer waiting time targets to be rolled out over the next five years. Specific cancer waiting times targets were set for 2001.
- Maximum one-month wait from urgent GP referral to treatment guaranteed for children's and testicular cancers and acute leukaemia.
- Maximum one-month wait from diagnosis to treatment for breast cancer.

Health Service Circular HSC 2001/012 (DH, 2001d)

Research shows that a top priority for patients is shorter waiting times. In response, the *Planning and Priorities Framework (PPF) – Mapping out the Priorities for Reform for the Next Three Years* promises concrete progress on reducing waits across the service. It aims to ensure that, by the end of 2008, no one waits more than 18 weeks from GP referral to hospital treatment.

(DH, 2004e)

Since the emphasis on targets for measuring the effectiveness of health care, there has been much debate about the way in which targets should be set and used as performance indicators. Campbell and Gibson (1997) summarise the desirable features of health targets as follows. They should:

- provide an overall goal and sense of purpose;
- be related to actions known to be effective;
- be achievable over a specified time;
- be realistic but challenging;
- be measurable and be able to be monitored;
- be agreed by those who have a part to play in their achievement;
- be expressed in terms of health improvements or reductions of risk factors to the population.

Activity

- Link these features to one of the targets described in the cancer plan.
- Consider whether these features can be linked to issues of kindness, compassion or empathy.
- How can targets be set for these characteristics of caring?

How can something like kindness or compassion be measured and how can we demonstrate their achievement within a specified timescale? This question raises issues about whether, within this managerialist approach to health care provision, the values of a humanistic approach to care will further diminish. It could be argued that a target-driven health care system, with the emphasis on performance indicators and measurement and resource allocation on the basis of target achievement, militates against the value of more qualitative aspects of care.

Resource allocation and professionalism

The issue of resource allocation can even determine the focus of the profession itself. As the NMC paper on the future role of nursing states (Longley *et al.*, 2008), one way of improving capacity in health care is role substitution, where the role is passed from one group of workers to another. As the technical imperative of health 'care' has expanded, so has the need for technically competent practitioners. Thus the professional role of nursing has expanded, with nurses engaging in more and more technical tasks.

Activity

List five or six technically focused skills that nurses now undertake that were undertaken only by medical staff 10–15 years ago.

Annandale (1998) suggests three reasons for the shift in boundaries between nursing and medicine.

1. It is cheaper for nurses to provide care than medical practitioners.
2. As a response to the New Deal for Junior Doctors (1991) and the European Working Time Directive (EWTD), a new contract for junior doctors was introduced in December 2000, requiring a statutory reduction in doctors' working hours. Since August 2001, it has been illegal for newly qualified junior doctors to work more than 56 hours per week or work without sufficient rest. The same standards have been applied to all doctors since August 2003. One way of offsetting this is to extend the role of nurses, so that they undertake some of the clinical tasks that junior doctors may have previously done. The introduction of nurse prescribing is a good example of this.
3. Nurses, Midwives and Health Visitors have undertaken professionalisation strategies, to improve their occupational status. Although the term 'profession' is sociologically contested (Johnson, 1972; Giddens, 2006), it is widely believed that a professional group displays a number of traits, including an exclusive body of knowledge, self-regulation and a governing body and an extended period of training (Greenwood, 1957). It has been argued that nursing has pursued a strategy of professionalisation through the acquisition of a unique body of theory, but also through the acquisition of skills that provide status (Gerrish *et al.*, 2003) and thus have focused on instrumental care at the expense of affective care (Peacock and Nolan, 2000).

Characteristics of a profession:
- systematic body of theory;
- professional authority;
- sanction of the community;
- regulatory code of ethics;
- the professional culture.

(Greenwood, 1957)

Activity

Using Greenwood's characteristics above, can nursing be viewed as a profession?

Transformations in health care and challenges to the biomedical model

Although there has been much emphasis on technological aspects of health care, and government and professional strategies have been developed to address the challenges of this, there is evidence that the nature of health care provision is changing. This provides opportunities for revisiting the concept of care and rebalancing affective care against instrumental care. The biomedical model is becoming increasingly challenged as the dominant framework for the delivery of health care in the twenty-first century. The changing demographics, improvements in living conditions and medical interventions have led to a change in the nature of dominant causes of morbidity and premature mortality. In the nineteenth century, acute infectious diseases were the major killers, but in the twenty-first century in the UK, chronic conditions are the major sources of morbidity. While there is a need for some medical intervention, the focus of health care has shifted from a curative focus to one of care and prevention.

Contemporary transformations in health and medicine

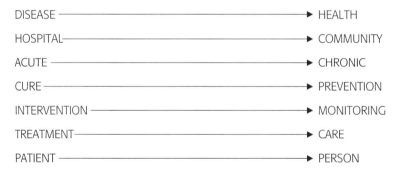

DISEASE ⟶ HEALTH

HOSPITAL ⟶ COMMUNITY

ACUTE ⟶ CHRONIC

CURE ⟶ PREVENTION

INTERVENTION ⟶ MONITORING

TREATMENT ⟶ CARE

PATIENT ⟶ PERSON

(Nettleton, 2006, p.11)

Activity

- Taking Nettleton's list above, describe one change in health care practice related to each individual transformation. For example, the focus on long-term conditions and self-care changes the focus of the disease of diabetes and its treatment. There is a shift from the focus on treatment where the doctor is the expert, to the expert patient, who lives with the disease in pursuit of optimum possible health.

This therefore raises questions about the continuing dominance of a technologically driven system of care and instrumental approach to caring. To some extent this was reflected in the NHS Performance Assessment Framework (1998) and the *Our Health, Our Care, Our Say* White Paper (DH, 2006a). Although many of the areas of health improvement remain focused on efficiency and outcomes, there is evidence that these transformations are being addressed through performance standards, with increased emphasis on health improvements and patient/user satisfaction.

NHS Performance Assessment Framework (1998) Areas
- Health improvement.
- Fair access.
- Effective delivery of appropriate health care.
- Efficiency.
- Patient/carer experience.
- Health outcomes of NHS care.

(Secretary of State for Health, 1998)

Our Health, Our Care, Our Say (DH, 2006a)
Three themes:
- putting people more in control of their own health and care;
- enabling and supporting health, independence and well-being;
- rapid and convenient access to high-quality, cost-effective care.

Four goals:
- better prevention services with earlier intervention;
- more choice and a louder voice (for people);
- more on tackling inequalities and improving access to community services;
- more support for people with long-term conditions.

(DH, 2006a)

There are also challenges within the health care division of labour. Although, historically, medicine has enjoyed superior status within this division of labour, the health care transformations have led to a shift in the balance of power. Patients and service users are becoming much more vocal in terms of consumer preferences, which in part reflects the political and ideological changes in health care, emphasising the importance of the consumer voice.

> There will be a radical and sustained shift in the way in which services are delivered – ensuring that they are more personalised

and that they fit into people's busy lives. We will give people a stronger voice so that they are the major drivers of service improvement.

(DH, 2006a)

In contemporary health care provision, there is a much stronger user and carer voice at every level of decision-making, and user views are sought in relation to aspects of care. Although much research demonstrates that patients still value the technical competent aspects of care (Morrison, 1991; Webb, 2001), there is also evidence of increased value being placed on affective and humanistic aspects of care in the late twentieth and early twenty-first centuries.

Complementary and alternative medicines (CAM)

The rise in the use of complementary and alternative medicines demonstrates a challenge to medicine's monopoly on health care provision, as people look for alternative sources of support. This may be associated with the changing nature of illness and Nettleton's representation of the transformation of health care as detailed above (Saks, 1994). In the absence of cures for long-term conditions, people may place more emphasis on care and humanistic components of health care. This is supported by Shumay *et al.* (2001), who evaluated the reasons why some people with cancer chose CAM instead of conventional medicine. The following were identified as reasons for people to choose CAM instead of conventional medicine.

- Participants reported negative interactions or missing communication with health care providers as being factors in their decision to decline conventional treatment.
- Participants reported positive or neutral interactions with health care providers regarding their use of CAM.

In an analysis of the concept of holism, Sarkis and Skoner (1987) identified two broad meanings within the nursing literature. Firstly, holism was understood in relation to the bio-psychosocial model of care, with nurses providing care that goes beyond the physical, encompassing more comprehensive needs, including cognitive and affective domains. Secondly, holistic care was conceptualised as incorporating care that was alternative to the traditional Western biomedical model, and included complementary and alternative approaches to health care. Nurses are increasingly incorporating these alternative methods into their practice. For example, Lynch (2007) describes the use of the emotional freedom technique, which is based on the ancient Chinese system of acupuncture (although it does not use needles) and is gaining popularity in the care of people who have had traumatic experiences. SAGA (2007) state that massage is the most commonly used alternative therapy for the relief of pain in people with cancer, and Liu and Fawcett (2008) discuss its use in relation to nursing practice.

Interpersonal relationships

Martin (1981) describes an expressive revolution in society generally, where people are much more publicly open about their emotions, and may seek outlets for the expression of these emotions. For example, there has been a burgeoning of counselling services, self-help groups and mutual support groups in many areas of life. While nurses are not counsellors (as discussed in Chapter 3), they may use counselling skills in the therapeutic encounter. However, the nurse will use interpersonal skills in all encounters with care recipients and, as argued throughout this book, many nursing paradigms, theories and models emphasise the centrality of the interpersonal relationship within good nursing practice. Therefore, nurses are ideally placed to respond to this wider change in society and use their education and skills to good effect in the provision of competent, compassionate and kind care. In a study of patient perceptions of the quality of care in high dependency units (HDUs), Brooks (1999) found that the patients placed value on technical skills, but also on the attitudes of the nursing staff. Positive statements about the caring nature of nursing staff included:

> 'Working from the heart – more than a job.'
> 'Dedicated nurse.'
> 'Staff bent over backwards to help you.'
>
> (Brooks, 1999, p. 332)

The value placed on caring skills

Although traditionally caring and emotional aspects of care have been undervalued, as argued in Chapter 1, there is growing evidence that this is being challenged. New social movements are a feature of the late twentieth and early twenty-first centuries, and have challenged the status quo of society's structures from a number of different perspectives. Feminism has been of particular importance, as feminists such as Pascall (1997) have questioned the gendered nature of caring and challenged the lack of value placed on women's caring skills. The result is that there is a shift in perceptions, with the act of caring being valued, not as an innate quality of the ideal woman (see Chapter 1), but as a skill which is valuable within the context of health care. This is reflected in the recognition of the care that is provided within the informal care sector, through legislation such as the Carers' Recognition Act 1995, but also in the increased recognition of the value of nursing. Nevertheless, despite the increased public popularity and perception of the value of nursing, pay differentials persist, with nurses' pay lagging behind those of comparable occupations (Waters, 2008). It seems there is still quite some way to go before the caring characteristics associated with nursing and gendered perceptions of femininity are truly valued and reflected in economic terms. Thus nurses continue to face the challenge of providing care in an environment that undervalues this humanistic value in financial terms.

Furthermore, the transformations in health care have led to an extension in the remit of caring. One of the features of contemporary health care policy is the shift from a focus on diagnosis, treatment and rehabilitation, to one on prevention of ill-health and health promotion as evidenced in successive policy documents from *The Health of the Nation* (DH, 1991b) through to *The NHS Plan* (DH, 2000) and *Our Health, Our Care, Our Say* (DH, 2006a). McKinlay (1979) uses the following analogy to describe the way that the biomedical framework focuses on illness, rather than the causes of illness:

> There I am standing by the shore of a swiftly flowing river and I hear the cry of a drowning man. So I jump into the river, put my arms around him, pull him to shore and apply artificial respiration. Just when he begins to breathe, there is another cry for help. So, I jump into the river, reach him, pull him to shore, apply artificial respiration, and then just as he begins to breathe, another cry for help. So back in the river again, without end, goes the sequence. You know, I am so busy jumping in, pulling them to shore, applying artificial respiration, that I have no time to see who the hell is upstream pushing them all in.

The new paradigm of health promotion and prevention of ill-health advocates a move away from this downstream focus, to one that focuses upstream to identify the causes of ill-health, whether they are located within the individual or within the wider social structures (Peterson and Waddell, 1998). This has implications for nursing care and the way that that care is focused. As a registered nurse, midwife or specialist community public health nurse, you must:

- protect and support the health of individual patients and clients;
- protect and support the health of the wider community;
- act in such a way that justifies the trust and confidence the public have in you;
- uphold and enhance the good reputation of the professions.

(NMC, 2004)

Care and the rationing of resources

Kendall (1992) argues that, historically, nursing has developed as a form of oppression, in that it has operated within the principles of the biomedical framework and dominant social structures. She argues that nursing practice has been concerned with a 'downstream' focus, where nurses have provided care within an illness-focused service, with the emphasis on individual adaptation and coping. However, this is not to say that care cannot be provided within this context and that the focus on downstream endeavours necessarily negates a humanistic focus. Indeed, Benner and Wrubel (1989) discuss the primacy of caring, arguing that caring is an essential element of helping people to cope.

> Because caring sets up what matters to a person, it also sets up what counts as stressful, and what options are available for coping. Caring creates possibility. This is the first way in which caring is primary.
>
> (Benner and Wrubel, 1989, p. 1)

Kendall argues that the focus on adaptation and coping results not only from the dual line of authority that traditional nursing has operated within, but also as a necessary response to a perceived lack of resources. As argued above, health care is costly and the rise in demand associated with demographic change, technological advances and consumers with access to a greater amount of information drives up demands and expectations, which cannot be matched by an associated rise in supply and provision of health care services. Thus rationing in health care is inevitable and is a continuing feature of contemporary health care (Hunter, 1997). Rationing decisions are constantly being made, in relation to types of treatments to be funded, populations or individuals who will have access to those treatments, as well as how money will be spent in relation to the health care workforce. In addition, nurses may find themselves faced with rationing decisions in relation to resources in terms of their time, where decisions have to be made about the most efficient way to spend the scarce resource of time. For Kendall, this has resulted in the prioritisation of care that fits in with the dominant paradigm of the biomedical model and the bureaucracy, which reinforces rules and regulations through decisions about the allocation of resources.

Activity

Thinking about the case studies used in this book, describe:
- two rationing decisions that were made by individual nurses;
- two rationing decisions that were made at an organisational level.

Emancipatory nursing practice

Kendall (1942), however, argues that the contemporary climate of health care allows nurses to be more proactive in the field of health promotion through what she terms emancipatory nursing practice. Emancipatory practice involves the liberation of care recipients, so that they are truly empowered to make decisions about their health care and, as such, emancipatory nursing practice has a political element. Moccia (1988) takes this a step further, arguing that social activism should be included as a component of care, as caring is undermined by the oppressive structures of poverty and inequality. How can nurses truly care for people if they continue to work within the structures and systems that deny people choices and freedoms in relation to their own health care? For example, consider the situation of a family who is living in poverty in a deprived area, with insufficient income to adequately provide all they need. They live in an overcrowded and damp house, without central heating, and the heating that they do have is inefficient because of ill-fitting windows. Both parents are unemployed and feel they have little prospect of finding long-term employment. This family has few choices about health. They may be able to make decisions about healthy diet, but even these are constrained by the situation that they find themselves in, as lifestyle choices are influenced by people's material and structural circumstances (Bunton *et al.*, 1995).

Thus, Kendall argues that nurses have a role to play in the preventative health care agenda, through challenging these societal inequalities that both contribute to illness and deny people the freedoms of choice about lifestyle and health care. For Kendall, critical understanding is a crucial element of emancipatory nursing action, and therefore nurse education has an important role to play in promoting emancipatory nursing practice.

Emancipatory nursing actions (critical awareness)
- Empowering self and others.
- Gaining critical awareness.
- Demonstrating power of critical knowledge.
- Understanding roots of oppression.
- Challenging status quo.
- Breaking barriers that keep one oppressed.

The role of nurse education

Mcilfatrick (2003) argues that a number of paradoxes face nurse education in the twenty-first century. Firstly, the demand for technological aspects of care and cure remains high, at the same time as there is a growing emphasis on health promotion and an expectation that nurses will take a lead in promoting health and well-being (DH, 1998). Secondly, there are public demands for greater professionalism in health care, and yet there is a growing emphasis on user and carer participation and lay assertiveness. The third paradox can be linked to the focus on competencies in pre-registration nursing programmes (UKCC, 1999). This has led to concerns about the relationship between technical competency and the qualities of caring, and a fear that caring may become sacrificed, with a focus on the achievement of technical competency. Thus there is a challenge for nurse educationalists to integrate education and training, so that nurses are competent and have the 'skills and ability to practise safely and effectively without the need for direct supervision' (UKCC, 1999), while also having the knowledge base (tacit, reflective, practical and experiential) to critically question practice and influence care and policy.

Within a process of critical reflection, contradictions between desirable work and actual practice are made visible and become the focus for action to resolve them. However, appropriate action may be difficult because of specific social norms and barriers (Mezirow, 1981) that are embodied within the fabric of the work environment. Indeed, the practitioner may feel powerless to take necessary action. It is in this sense that the practitioner needs both challenge and support to confront practices as exposed through reflection on experience (Johns, 1995). Nurse education is therefore crucial in developing this critical awareness and critical knowledge, so as to adequately provide nurses with the skills and confidence to be proactive change agents in a dynamic health and social care system.

Caring and stress

Caring is also stressful, involving an emotional labour and challenging people's sense of self. Bolton (2000) argues that the emotional work of caring is increasingly being recognised, but that it is physically hard and needs to be valued in the same way that physical and technical labour is valued. Benner and Wrubel (1989) identified stress and burnout associated with caring work, and the fact that a major contributing factor is the societal undervaluing of this work. Burnout is a negative psychological consequence of depersonalisation, reduced sense of personal achievement and emotional exhaustion (Maslach, 1982). In addition, nurses are often working with people who are experiencing vulnerability and may offer emotional work as a gift, which then involves them in an emotional situation. At the same time, nurses are required to suppress their own emotions in order to be able to facilitate coping in others. Thus nurses' sense of personal knowledge and security may be under threat as they engage in a caring relationship. This therefore underlines the importance of personal knowledge as defined by Carper (1978), as well as a need for nurses themselves to have supportive networks, and the ability to reflect, learn and challenge existing systems and ideas.

Heath (1998) identifies the importance of reflection in the development of expert practitioners (Benner, 1984) as the process of reflection is used as a transformational learning tool, where nurses reflect on theory and practice and bridge the theory/practice gap to develop a knowledge for practice, which helps in the pursuit of proficiency, competency and expert nursing actions. In a study of nurses' perceptions of reflective learning, Burnard (1995) found that many nurses felt that reflection helped them to improve on their practice:

> I think it makes you a more confident practitioner and a more competent practitioner. It makes you a more sensitive practitioner as well. It gives you the opportunity to look at your practice and improve on it.

The twenty-first century is characterised by a continuum of health care – the need for cures and treatment associated with the technological imperatives remains but, at the same time, there is growing emphasis on health promotion, with strategies for prevention and health surveillance (Armstrong, 2004). Nurses need therefore to have a strong foundation of knowledge in Carper's four dimensions of knowing, to equip them with the personal confidence and value system and evidence base to provide good-quality care that is ethically sound and demonstrates both technical and aesthetic competence and challenges the deficiencies in the health care system. White (1995) adds a further dimension of nursing knowledge, arguing that nurses need to have socio-political knowing, since health care work is situated in and influenced by political, social and economic context. Social scientific knowledge is therefore seen as important to the development of nursing professionals with the critical skills to influence patient care and health care policy (Porter and Ryan, 1996; White, 1995). For White, it is not just organisational constraints and scarce resources that impact on nursing practice, but also the issues of power (see Chapter 6). Power in health care and the health care division of labour is important in relation to who has influence over policy, sets of ideas and resources (Heath, 1998). If nurses want to have their voices heard, then critical questions need to be asked about these issues of power. Knowledge is power, and nurses are ideally placed to use their knowledge base and critical thinking skills to unharness their power and reassert the primacy of caring and the value of every aspect of care in contemporary health care practice.

Burton (2000) questions whether nurses are ready to confront these issues of power and take on the demands of critical thinking and emancipatory practice. However, there is evidence that reflective learning can help nurses to develop skills and abilities to empathise with others, while at the same time challenging the status quo (Conway, 1998; Platzer *et al.*; 2000).

THE FUTURE

Fagerstrom *et al.*'s (1998) analysis of care is useful for summarising the position of care in contemporary health care practice. They identified three deficiencies in the health care system, which may lead to people feeling insufficiently cared for:

- deficiency in the system, where nurses have excessive workload and so do not have time to care;
- deficiency in the caring culture, where the focus of caring today is on identifying symptoms, on illness and its treatment;
- caring deficiency, where the patient does not feel noticed and understood and will to some extent suffer pain unnecessarily or suffer loneliness.

The challenges of the future are multiple and not easy to overcome, but nurses are ideally placed to use their knowledge and skills to good effect in promoting changes in health care practice in the twenty-first century. There are a growing number of media stories and anecdotes about poor-quality care (de Reybekill, 2008) and nurses need to find a way to redress this balance, not only in challenging these mass media messages, but also in reasserting the primacy of caring and valuing all aspects of the unique role of nursing. This is especially challenging, as nursing takes place in a bureaucratic system of health care, with emphasis on efficiency and cost containment. However, unless nurses articulate the value of caring within the wider organisation of health care, there is a danger that caring will continue to be devalued (Peacock and Nolan, 2000). Sourial (1997) argues that caring needs to be seen within a broader context than the individual nurse–patient relationship, with structural factors affecting the function of caring. She uses Valentine's (1989) work to argue that nurses should define what is meant by caring and identify the fact that:

> The availability of resources to support the caring interaction also affects the quality of that relationship.
> (Valentine, 1989, p. 30, cited by Sourial, 1997)

In a cost-driven health care system, nurses need to articulate the benefits of care to the enhancement of quality care and improved patient outcomes.

The impact that a nurse's caring can have on a patient is not mentioned in conversations about health care systems and is not measurable by any known tool. And yet that impact is profoundly powerful: It is the invisible power of nursing . . . The choice to care, and to express that care and compassion by our behaviour is the absolutely correct choice nurses must make in order to continue serving society justly.

(Manthey, 2008, p. 4)

SUMMARY

- Nursing and caring do not operate in a vacuum, but are influenced by the social, political and economic system of which they are a part.
- Contemporary health care transformations provide an opportunity for the re-evaluation of care and the re-emphasis on humanistic and qualitative aspects of caring.
- Nurse education has an important role to play in developing nurses who have the knowledge, skills and confidence to provide good instrumental and affective care to care recipients.
- Nurses need to take ownership of the concept of care and use their knowledge and skills to articulate its importance within health care.

FURTHER READING

Bradshaw, P.L. and Bradshaw, G. (2004) *Health policy for health care professionals*. London: Sage
This is a useful contemporary guide to the health service, which is tailored specifically to the exploration of challenges that health care professionals may encounter.

Kendall, J. (1992) 'Fighting back: promoting emancipatory nursing actions'. *Advances in Nursing Science*, 15(2): 1–15
This is an interesting article that challenges the reader to think about nursing practice and the role of nurses in enabling people to make choices about health and health care.

Nettleton, S. (2006) *Sociology of health and illness* (2nd ed.). Cambridge: Polity Press
This book is an accessible text that provides a critical discussion of the historical development of the biomedical model and the contemporary transformations in health care.

Peacock, J.W. and Nolan, P.W. (2000) 'Care under threat in the modern world'. *Journal of Advanced Nursing*, 32(5): 1066–70
This article provides a useful summary of the historical development of nursing and the concept of care, highlighting ways in which care needs to be articulated by nurses in the twenty-first century.

Appendix 1

THE NMC ESSENTIAL SKILLS CLUSTERS

(Adapted from the NMC Guidance for the Introduction of the Essential Skills Clusters for Pre-registration Nursing Programmes, Annex 1 to NMC Circular 07/2007.)

The NMC has a duty under the Nursing and Midwifery Order 2001 to set standards for education programmes and to keep these under review. For pre-registration nursing these are set out within *The Standards of Proficiency for Pre-registration Nursing Education* (NMC, 2004) (Nursing Standards). The introduction of the NMC Essential Skills Clusters (ESCs) supports the achievement of the Nursing Standards and are mandatory for all pre-registration nursing.

The Skills Clusters were developed as an outcome of the review of fitness for practice at the point of registration and aim to provide clarity of expectation for the public and profession alike to complement the existing NMC pre-registration outcomes and proficiencies for better ensuring entry to the branch programme and subsequently to the register, so that new qualifiers are capable of safe and effective practice. The need for a progression point between the Common Foundation Programme and a branch area was reinforced.

The ESCs are UK-wide generic skills statements set out under broad headings that identify skills to support the achievement of the existing NMC outcomes for entry to the branch, and the proficiencies for entry to the register. These Nursing Standards continue to exist and are unchanged. The ESCs are generic and applicable to all four branches of nursing. Those identified for entry to the register should be addressed within the context of the branch field of practice. The focus has been on identifying skills that are essential rather than identifying all component skills relating to a specific area of practice. The clusters do not encompass all the skills needed to be proficient as a nurse; what they do is to address potential areas of deficit so that the public can be assured that they are identified and assessed within every pre-registration nursing programme across the UK. ESCs are being introduced for:

- care and compassion;
- communication;
- organisational aspects of care;
- infection prevention and control;
- nutrition and fluid maintenance;
- medicines management.

To download the Essential Skills Clusters please visit:
www.nmc-uk.org/aArticle.aspx?ArticleID=2914

Appendix 2

THE NHS KNOWLEDGE AND SKILLS FRAMEWORK

(Adapted from *The NHS Knowledge and Skills Framework* document, DH, 2004a.)

The NHS Knowledge and Skills Framework (the NHS KSF) defines and describes the knowledge and skills that NHS staff need to apply in their work in order to deliver quality services. It provides a single, consistent, comprehensive and explicit framework on which to base review and development for all staff.

The purpose of the NHS KSF is to facilitate the development of services so that they better meet the needs of users and the public through investing in the development of all members of staff. The NHS KSF is based on the principles of good people management – how people like to be treated at work and how organisations can enable people to work effectively. It supports the effective learning and development of individuals and teams, with all members of staff being supported to learn throughout their careers and develop in a variety of ways, and being given the resources to do so. It supports the development of individuals in the post in which they are employed so that they can be effective at work, with managers and staff being clear about what is required within a post and managers enabling staff to develop within their post. It promotes equality for and diversity of all staff, with every member of staff using the same framework, having the same opportunities for learning and development open to them and having the same structured approach to learning, development and review.

The NHS KSF is about the application of knowledge and skills – not about the specific knowledge and skills that individuals need to possess. As a broad generic framework it is designed to be applicable and transferable across the NHS and to draw out the general aspects that show how individuals need to apply their knowledge and skills within the NHS. It is a broad generic framework that focuses on the application of knowledge and skills – it does not describe the exact knowledge and skills that people need to develop. The NHS KSF is designed to form the basis of a development review process. This is an ongoing cycle of review, planning, development and evaluation for all staff in the NHS which links organisational and individual development needs – a commitment to the development of everyone who works in the NHS.

The NHS KSF is made up of 30 dimensions. The dimensions identify broad functions that are required by the NHS to enable it to provide a good-quality service to the public. Six of these dimensions are core, which means that they are relevant to every post in the NHS. The core dimensions are:

1. Communication.
2. Personal and people development.
3. Health, safety and security.
4. Service improvement.
5. Quality.
6. Equality and diversity.

The other 24 dimensions are specific – they apply to some but not all jobs in the NHS. The specific dimensions are grouped into themes as shown below but will not be mapped within this book.

- Health and well-being.
- Estates and facilities.
- Information and knowledge.
- General.

For further information see *The NHS Knowledge and Skills Framework* (NHS KSF) and the *Development Review Process* (DH, 2004a):
**www.dh.gov.uk/en/Publicationsandstatistics/Publications/
PublicationsPolicyAndGuidance/DH_4090843**

Appendix 3

THE ESSENCE OF CARE: PATIENT-FOCUSED BENCHMARKING FOR HEALTH CARE PRACTITIONERS

(Adapted from *The essence of care: patient-focused benchmarking for health care practitioners*, (DH, 2001a))

The NHS Plan (DH, 2000) reinforced the importance of 'getting the basics right' and of improving the patient experience. *The Essence of Care* (DH, 2001), launched in February 2001, provides a tool to help practitioners take a patient-focused and structured approach to sharing and comparing practice. It has enabled health care personnel to work with patients to identify best practice and to develop action plans to improve care.

Patients, carers and professionals worked together to agree and describe good-quality care and best practice. This resulted in benchmarks covering eight areas of care.

- Continence and bladder and bowel care.
- Personal and oral hygiene.
- Food and nutrition.
- Pressure ulcers.
- Privacy and dignity.
- Record-keeping.
- Safety of clients with mental health needs in acute mental health and general hospital settings.
- Principles of self-care.

Two subsequent benchmarks were added, covering:

- Promoting health.
- The care environment.

This document containing the toolkit for benchmarking the fundamentals of care including the background to *Essence of Care*, a description of the benchmarking tool, how to use the benchmarks, and record forms for developing action and business plans can be downloaded from: **www.dh.gov.uk/en/Publicationsandstatistics/Publications/ PublicationsPolicyAndGuidance/DH_4005475**

References

Action on Smoking and Health (2007) Stopping smoking: the benefits and aids to quitting. **www.ash.org.uk/files/documents/ASH_116. pdf** (23/5/08)

Action on Smoking and Health (2008) Facts at a glance **www.ash. org.uk/files/ documents/ASH_93.pdf** (23/5/08)

Allen, D. and Hughes, D. (2002) *Nursing and the division of labour in health care.* London: Palgrave MacMillan

Allen, J. (2000) 'Power; its institutional guises (and disguises)' in Hughes, G. and Fergusson, R. (eds) *Ordering lives: family work and welfare.* London: Routledge

Allmark, P. (1998) 'Is caring a virtue?' *Journal of Advanced Nursing,* 28(3): 466–72

Allsop, J. (1984) *Health policy and the National Health Service.* London: Longman

Annandale, E. (1998) *The sociology of health and medicine: a critical introduction.* Cambridge: Polity Press

Annual Report of the Chief Medical Officer (1973) *On the State of the Public Health.* London: HMSO

Antonovsky, A. (1987) *Unravelling the mystery of health, how people manage stress and stay well.* San Francisco: Jossey-Bass

Argyris, C. (1991) 'Teaching smart people to learn'. *Reflections,* 4 (2). **www. velinperformance.com/downloads/chris_argyris_learning.pdf** (23/5/08)

Argyris, C. and Schön, D. (1974) *Theory in practice: increasing personal effectiveness.* Massachusetts: Addison-Wesley

Armstrong, D. (2004) 'The rise of surveillance medicine', in Annandale, E., Elston, M.A. and Prior, L. (eds) *Medical work, medical knowledge and health care.* Oxford: Blackwell

Audit Commission (2002) *Forget me not 2002: developing mental health services for older people in England.* 21 Feb 2002. Wetherby: Audit Commission

Baillie, L. (ed.) (2001) *Practical nursing skills.* London: Arnold

Baines, C., Evans, P. and Neysmith, S.N. (eds) (1991) *Women's caring: feminist perspectives on social welfare.* Toronto: McClelland and Stewart

Ball, J. and Pike, G. (2005) *Managing to work differently.* Royal College of Nursing and Employment Research

Becze, E. (2007) 'Learn to be sensitive to patients' cultural differences'. *ONS Connect,* November, 2007, p31

Benner, P. (1984) *From novice to expert.* California: Addison-Wesley

Benner, P. and Wrubel, J. (1989) *The primacy of caring.* New York: Addison Wesley

Benner, P., Tanner, C. and Chesla, C. (1996) *Expertise in nursing practice*. New York: Springer

Bjork, I.T. (1999) 'Practical skills development in new nurses'. *Nursing Inquiry*, 6: 34–47

Blank, R.H. and Merrick, J.A. (2005) *End-of-life decision making*. Cambridge, Mass.: MIT Press

Bolton, S. (2000) 'Who cares? Offering emotion work as a "gift" in the nursing labour process'. *Journal of Advanced Nursing*, 32(3): 580–6

Bonham, P. (2004) *Communicating as a mental health carer*. Cheltenham: Nelson Thornes

Boreham, R., Airey, C., Erens, B. and Tobin, R. (National Centre for Social Research) for the Department of Health (2003) National surveys of NHS patients: General practice, 2002. **www.dh.gov.uk/en/Publicationsandstatistics/Publications/PublicationsStatistics/DH_4119 522**

Boud, D., Keough, R., and Walker, D. (1985) *Reflection: turning experience into learning*. London: Kogan Page

Boyd, E.M. and Fales, A.W. (1983) 'Reflective learning key to learning from experience'. *Journal of Humanistic Psychology*, 23(2): 99–117

Boykin, A. and Schoenhofer, S. (1991) 'Story as the link between nursing practice, ontology, and epistemology'. *Journal of Nursing Scholarship*, 23(4): 245–8

Bradbury, M. (1998) *Representations of death: a social psychological perspective*. London: Routledge

Brager, G. and Specht, H. (1973) *Community organising*. Columbia: Columbia University Press

Brilowski, G.A. and Wendler, M. (2005) 'An evolutionary concept of caring'. *Journal of Advanced Nursing*, 50(6): 641–50

Brooks, N. (1999) 'Patients' perspective of quality of care in a high-dependency unit'. *Intensive and Critical Care Nursing*, 15: 324–37

Brotherton, G. and Parker, S. (2008) *Your foundation in health and social care*. London: Sage

Bunton, R., Nettleton, S. and Burrows, R. (eds) (1995) *The sociology of health promotion: critical analyses of consumption, lifestyle and risk*. London: Routledge

Burnard, P. (1990) *Learning human skills: an experiential guide for nurses* (2nd ed.). Oxford: Butterworth-Heinemann

Burnard, P. (1992) *Communicate!* London: Edward Arnold

Burnard, P. (1994) *Effective communication skills for health professionals*. London: Chapman and Hall

Burnard, P. (1995) 'Nurse educators' perceptions of reflection and reflective practice: a report of a descriptive study'. *Journal of Advanced Nursing*, 21: 1167–74

Burnard, P. (1999) *Counselling skills for health professionals*. Cheltenham: Stanley Thornes

Burton, A.J. (2000) 'Reflection: nursing's practice and education panacea?' *Journal of Advanced Nursing*, 31: 1009–17

Campbell, H. and Gibson, A. (1997) 'Health targets in the NHS: lessons learned from experience with breast feeding targets in Scotland', *BMJ* 314:1030 (5 April)

Capuzzo, M., Laundi, F., Bassani, A., Grassi, L., Vlta, C. and Alvisa, R. (2005) 'Emotional and interpersonal factors are most important for patient satisfaction with anesthesia'. *Acta Anaesthesiol. Scand*, 49: 735–42

Carper, B. (1978) 'Fundamental ways of knowing in nursing'. *Advances in Nursing Science*, 1(1): 13–23

Carr, S. (2000) 'The comfort of small things'. *Health Service Journal*, 16 March: 31

Chang, S.O. (2001) 'The conceptual structure of physical touch in caring'. *Journal of Advanced Nursing*, 33(6): 820–7

Chinn, P.L. and Kramer, M.K. (1995) *Theory and nursing: a systematic approach* (4th ed.). St Louis: Mosby

Chooporian, T. (1986) 'Reconceptualizing the environment', in Moccia, P. op cit.

Clamp, C. (1980) 'Learning through incidents'. *Nursing Times*, 76(40): 1755–8

Clarke, A. (2001) *The sociology of healthcare*. London: Prentice Hall

Commission for Social Care Inspection (2007) *Rights, risks and restraints*. 17 December 2007. London: CSCI

Conway, J.E. (1998) 'Evolution of the species "expert nurse". An examination of the practical knowledge held by expert nurses'. *Journal of Clinical Nursing*, 7: 75–82

Cooper, M.C. (1991) 'Principle oriented ethics and the ethics of care: a creative tension'. *Advances in Nursing Science*, 14(2): 22–31

Cross, T., Bazron, B., Dennis, K., and Isaacs, M. (1989) *Toward a culturally competent system of care*. Vol. 1. Washington, D.C.: Georgetown University

Curzon, L. (1990) *Teaching in further education*. New York: Holt, Rinehart and Winston

Daily Telegraph (2007) 'Veteran "treated like a parcel" by nursing home staff'. 15 December 2007

Daley, J., Speedy, S., Jackson, D. and Darbyshire, P. (eds) (2002) *Contexts of nursing: an introduction*. Oxford: Blackwell

Dalley, G. (1988) *Ideologies of caring: rethinking community and collectivism*. Basingstoke: Macmillan

Davies, B. and O'Berle, K. (1990) 'Dimensions of the supportive role of the nurse in palliative care'. *Oncology Nurses Forum*, 17: 87–94

Davies, C. (1995) *Gender and the professional predicament in nursing*. Buckingham: Open University Press

Department of Health (1989) *Working for patients*. London: HMSO

Department of Health (1991a) *The patients charter*. London: HMSO

Department of Health (1991b) *The health of the nation*. London: HMSO

Department of Health (1992) *Meeting the spiritual needs of patients and staff*. HSG(92) 2. Health Service Guidelines. London: NHS Management Executive

Department of Health (1997) *The new NHS: modern, dependable*. London: HMSO

Department of Health (1998) *Independent inquiry into inequalities in health* (Acheson Report). London: HMSO

Department of Health (2000) *The NHS Plan.* London: HMSO

Department of Health (2001a) *The essence of care: patient-focused benchmarking for health care practitioners.* London: HMSO

Department of Health (2001b) *The expert patient: a new approach to chronic disease management for the 21st century.* London: HMSO

Department of Health (2001c) *Your guide to the NHS: getting the most from your National Health Service.* London: HMSO

Department of Health (2001d) Health Service Circular (HSC) 2001/012. *Achieving the NHS cancer plan waiting time targets.* London: HMSO

Department of Health (2002a) *Whose hands on your genes?* London: HMSO

Department of Health (2002b) *Mental health policy implementation guide.* London: HMSO

Department of Health (2004a) *The NHS knowledge and skills framework.* London: HMSO

Department of Health (2004b) *NHS improvement plan.* London: HMSO

Department of Health (2004c) *Choosing health.* White Paper. London: HMSO

Department of Health (2004d) *4-hour checklist: reducing delays for A & E patients.* London: HSMO

Department of Health (2004e) *National standards, local action: health and social care standards and planning framework 2005/06–2007/08.* London: HMSO

Department of Health (2005a) *Now I feel tall.* London: HMSO

Department of Health (2005b) *Creating a patient-led NHS.* London: HMSO

Department of Health (2005c) *National service framework for long term conditions.* London: HMSO

Department of Health (2006a) *Our health, our care, our say.* London: HMSO

Department of Health (2006b) *Dignity in care.* London: HMSO

Department of Health (2006c) *Modernising nursing careers – setting the direction.* London: HMSO

Department of Health (2006d) *Essence of care benchmarks for promoting health.* London: HMSO

Department of Health (2007a) *Essence of care: benchmarks for the care environment.* London: HMSO

Department of Health (2007b) *Commissioning a brighter future. Improving access to psychological therapies: positive practice guide.* London: HMSO

Department of Health, Social Services and Public Safety (1998) *Valuing diversity: a way forward: a strategy for nursing, midwifery and health visiting.* Belfast: The Stationery Office

De Reybekill, N. (2008) 'Trust me . . . I'm a modern health care professional'. *Health Service Journal,* 17 April 2008: 16–17

Dewey, J. (1933) *How we think.* Boston: D. C. Heath

Dex, S. (1985) *The sexual division of work: conceptual revolutions in the social sciences.* Brighton: Harvester Wheatsheaf

Donabedian, A. (1966) in Al-Assaf, M.D. and Schmele, R.N. (1993) *The text book of total quality in healthcare.* Florida: St Lucie Press

Duffin, C. (2008) 'Brushing up on oral hygiene'. *Nursing Older People*, 20(2): 14–16

Edwards, S. (1998) 'An anthropological interpretation of nurses' and patients' perceptions of the use of space and touch'. *Journal of Advanced Nursing*, 28(4): 809–17

Egan, G. (2002) *The skilled helper* (7th ed.). Pacific Grove, CA: Brooks/Cole

Eisenburg, N. and Miller, P. (1987) in Omdahl, B. and O'Donnel, C. (1999) 'Emotional, contagion, empathetic concern and communicative responsiveness as variables affecting nurses' stress and occupational commitment'. *Journal of Advanced Nursing*, 29 (6): 1351–9

Ekebergh, M., Lepp, M. and Dahlburgh, K. (2004) 'Reflective learning with drama'. *Nurse Education Today*, 24(8): 622–8

Eriksson, K. (1994) in Fagerström, L., Eriksson, K. and Bergbom Endberg, I. (1998) 'The patient's caring needs as a message of suffering'. *Journal of Advanced Nursing*, 28 (5): 978–87

Ersser, S.J. (1998) The presentation of the nurse: a neglected dimension of therapeutic nurse–patient interaction', in McMahon, R. and Pearson, A. *Nursing as therapy*. Cheltenham: Stanley Thornes

Escudero-Carretero, M., Prieto-Rodriguez, A., Fernandez-Fernandez, I. and March-Cerda, J. (2007) 'Expectations held by type 1 and 2 diabetes mellitus patients and their relatives'. *Health Expectations*, 10: 337–49

Fagerström, L., Eriksson, K. and Bergbom Endberg, I. (1998) 'The patient's caring needs as a message of suffering'. *Journal of Advanced Nursing*, 28 (5): 978–87

Fealy, G.M. (1995) 'Professional caring: the moral dimension'. *Journal of Advanced Nursing*, 22(6): 1135–40

Finch, J. and Groves, D. (1983) *A labour of love: women, work and caring*. London: Routledge and Kegan Paul

Flanagan, J. (1954) 'The critical incident technique'. *Psychological Bulletin*, 51: 327–58

Fosbinder, D. (1994) 'Patient perceptions of nursing care: an emerging theory of interpersonal competence'. *Journal of Advanced Nursing*, 20: 1085–93

Fredriksson, L. (1999) 'Modes of relating in a caring conversation: a research synthesis on presence touch and listening'. *Journal of Advanced Nursing*, 30(5): 1167–78

Fredriksson, L. and Lindstrom, U.A. (2002) 'Caring conversations – psychiatric patients' narratives about suffering'. *Journal of Advanced Nursing*, 40(4): 396–404

Freshwater, D. (ed.) (2002) *Therapeutic nursing: improving patient care through self awareness and reflection*. London: Sage

Freud, S. (1936) *The problem of anxiety*. New York: W.W. Norton

Fry, S.T. (1991) 'A theory of caring: pitfalls and promises', in Gaut, D.A. and Leininger, M.M. (eds) *Caring: the compassionate healer*. New York: National League for Nursing

Geissler, P. and McCord, F. (1986) 'Dental care in the elderly'. *Nursing Times*, 82(20): 53–4

Gerrish, K., McManus, M. and Ashworth, P. (2003) 'Creating what sort of professional? Master's level nurse education as a professionalizing strategy'. *Nursing Inquiry*, 10(2): 103–12

Gibbs, G. (1988) *Learning by doing: a guide to teaching and learning methods.* Oxford: Oxford Brooks University

Giddens, A. (1991) *Modernity and self-identity: self and society in the late modern age.* Cambridge: Polity Press

Giddens, A. (2006) *Sociology* (5th ed.). Cambridge: Polity Press

Gillon, R. (1994) 'Medical ethics: four principles plus attention to scope'. *British Medical Journal*, 1994:184–8

Gladwell, M. (2005) *Blink. The power of thinking without thinking.* Washington: Time Warner Books

Goff, S. (1999) 'Towards the end of life: dying and death, transcendence and legacies', in Heath, H. and Schofield, I. *Healthy ageing: nursing older people.* London: Mosby

Gomm, R. and Davies, C. (eds) (2000) *Using evidence in health and social care.* Buckingham: Open University Press

Gould, N. (2004) *Social work, critical reflection and the learning organisation.* Aldershot: Ashgate

Gournay, K. and Brooking, J. (1995) 'The community psychiatric nurse in primary care: an economic analysis'. *Journal of Advanced Nursing*, 22: 769–78

Gove, P.B. (1986) in Brilowski and Wendler (2005) 'An evolutionary concept of caring'. *Journal of Advanced Nursing*, 50(6): 641–50

Graham, H. (1983) 'Caring: a labour of love', in Finch, J. and Groves, D. (eds) *A labour of love: women, work and caring.* London: Routledge and Kegan Paul

Graham, H. (1993) *When life's a drag.* London: Department of Health

Green, C. (2002) 'Reflections on reflection: students' evaluation of their moving and handling education'. *Nurse Education in Practice*, 2: 4–12

Greenwood, E. (1957) 'Attributes of a profession'. *Social Work*, 2(3): 44–55

Gretta, L. (1893) The Nightingale pledge. **www.accd.edu/sac/nursing/honors. html** (23/5/08)

Griffiths, J. and Boyle, S. (2005) *Holistic oral care: a guide for health professionals.* London: Stephen Hancocks Ltd.

Gropper, E.I. (1992) 'Promoting health by promoting comfort'. *Nursing Forum*, 27 (5): 8

Hallsdorsdottir, S. and Hamrin, E. (1997) 'Caring and uncaring encounters within nursing and healthcare from the cancer patient's perspective'. *Cancer Nursing*, 20 (2): 120–8

Ham, C. (1999) *Health policy in Britain* (4th ed.). Basingstoke: Macmillan

Hardey, M. (1999) 'Doctor in the house: the internet as a source of lay health knowledge and the challenge to expertise'. *Sociology of Health and Illness*, 21(6)

Healthcare Commission (2004) *Standards for better health.* London: HMSO

Healthcare Commission (2007) *Caring for dignity: a national report on dignity in care for older people while in hospital.* London: HMSO

Health Protection Agency, Institute of Child Health, Islington PCT and Great Ormond Street Hospital, Department of Health (2005) *National minmum standards for immunisation training.* London: HMSO

Heath, H. (1998) 'Reflection and patterns of knowing in nursing'. *Journal of Advanced Nursing,* 27: 1054–9

Henderson, V.A. (1991) *The nature of nursing. Reflections after 25 years.* New York: National League for Nursing

Henderson, A. (2001) 'Emotional labour and nursing: an under-appreciated aspect of caring work'. *Nursing Inquiry,* 8(2): 130–8

Heron, J. (2001) *Helping the client* (5th ed.). London: Sage

Hochschild, A.R. (1983) *The managed heart: commercialization of human feelings.* Berkeley, CA: California University Press

Hogston, R. and Marjoram, B.A. (2007) F*oundations of nursing practice: leading the way.* Basingstoke: Palgrave Macmillan

Holland, M. (2004) 'Patient stories'. *Nursing Standard,* November 3(8): 21

Hunter, D. (1997) *Desperately seeking solutions: rationing health care.* London: Longman

Huycke, L. and All, A. (2000) 'Quality in health care and ethical principles'. *Journal of Advanced Nursing,* 32(3): 562–71

James, N. (1989) 'Emotional labour: skill and work in the social regulation of feelings'. *Sociological Review,* 31(1): 15–42

Jasper, M. (1999) in Scholes, J., Webb, C., Gray, M., Endacott, R., Miller, C., Jasper, M. and McMulan, M. (2004) 'Making portfolios work in practice'. *Journal of Advanced Nursing,* 46(6): 595–603

Johns, C. (1995) 'Framing learning through refection within Carper's fundamental ways of knowing in nursing'. *Journal of Advanced Nursing,* 22: 226–34

Johns, C. (2002) *Guided reflection: advancing practice.* Oxford: Blackwell

Johnson, D.E. (1980) 'The behavioural system model for nursing', in Riehl, J. P. and Roy, C. (eds) *Conceptual models for nursing practice.* New York: Appleton-Century-Crofts

Johnson, T. (1972) *Professions and power.* London: Macmillan

Jones, L. and Sidell, M. (eds) (1997) *The challenges of promoting health.* Buckingham: Open University Press

Jossens, M.O. and Ganley, B.J. (2006) 'Integrated health practices: development of a graduate nursing program'. *Journal of Nursing Education,* 45(1): 16–24

Kellehear, A. (1990) *Dying of cancer: the final year of life.* London: Harwood Academic

Kendall, J. (1992) 'Fighting back: promoting emancipatory nursing actions'. *Advances in Nursing Science,* 15(2): 1–15

Kershaw, B. and Salvage, J. (eds) (1986) *Models for nursing.* Kings Lynn: J Wiley and Sons

King, I.M. (1981) *A theory for nursing: systems, concepts, process.* New York: John Wiley and Sons

Kitwood, T. (1997) *Dementia reconsidered: the person comes first.* Buckingham: Open University Press

Klein, R. (1995) *The new politics of the NHS* (3rd ed.) London: Longman

Kubler-Ross, E. (1970) *On death and dying.* New York: MacMillan

Lawler, J. (1991) *Behind the scenes: nursing, somology and the problem of the body*. London: Churchill Livingstone

Leininger, M.M. (1980) 'Caring: A central focus for nursing and health care services'. *Nursing and Health Care*, 176: 135–43

Leininger, M.M. (1991) *Culture, care, diversity and universality: a theory of nursing*. New York: National League of Nursing Press

Leininger, M.M. (1995) *Transcultural nursing: concepts, theories, research and practice* (2nd ed.). New York: McGraw-Hill

Lewis, G. (ed.) (1998) *Forming nation, framing welfare*. London: Routledge in association with Open University Press

Lindberg, J.B., Love Hunter, M. and Kruszewski, A. (1990) *Introduction to nursing: concepts, issues and opportunities*. Philadelphia: Lippincott

Littlewood, J. (1992) *Aspects of grief: bereavement in adult life*. London: Routledge

Liu, Y. and Fawcett, T.N. (2008) 'The role of massage therapy in the relief of cancer pain'. *Nursing Standard*, 22 (21): 35–40

Longley, M., Shaw C. and Dolan, G. (2007) *Nursing towards 2015*. Pontypridd: Welsh Institute for Health and Social Care

Lynch, E. (2007) 'Emotional acupuncture'. *Nursing Standard*, 21(50): 24–5

Macionis, J. and Plummer, K. (2005) *Sociology: a global introduction* (3rd ed.). Harlow: Prentice Hall

Mallik, M. (1997) 'Advocacy in nursing: a review of the literature'. *Journal of Advanced Nursing*, 25: 130–8

Mangen, S.P., Paykell, E.S., Griffith, J.H., Buxhell, A. and Mancini, P. (1983) 'Cost-effectiveness of community psychiatric nurse or out-patient psychiatrist care'. *Medicine*, 33: 407–16

Manley, K. and Garbett, B. (2000) 'Paying Peter and Paul: reconciling concepts of expertise with competency for clinical career structure', *Journal of Clinical Nursing*, 9: 347–59

Manthey, M. (2008) 'The invisible power of nursing'. *Creative Nursing*, 14(1): '3–5

Martin, B. (1981) *A sociology of contemporary change*. Oxford: Blackwell

Martin, R.A. (2006) *The psychology of humour: an integrative approach*. London: Elsevier

Maslach, C. (1982) *Burnout: The cost of caring*. Englewood Cliffs, NJ: Prentice Hall

Maslow, A. (1954) *Motivation and personality*. New York: Harper and Row

Maslow, A. (1962) *Towards a psychology of being*. New York: Harper and Row

McCance, T.V., McKenna, H.P. and Boore, J.R.P. (1999) 'Caring: theoretical perspectives of relevance to nursing'. *Journal of Advanced Nursing*, 30(6): 1388–95

McClymont, M. (1999) 'Health and wellness', in Heath, H. and Schofield, I. *Healthy ageing: nursing older people*. London: Mosby

McCorkle, R. (1974) 'Effects of touch on seriously ill patients'. *Nursing Research*, 23: 125–32

McCreaddie, M. and Wiggins, S. (2008) 'The purpose and function of humour and health care and nursing: a narrative review'. *Journal of Advanced Nursing*, 61(6) 584–95

Mcilfatrick, S. (2004) 'The future of nurse education: characterised by paradoxes'. *Nurse Education Today*, 24: 79–83

McKinlay, J.B. (1979) 'A case for refocusing upstream; the political economy of illness', in E.G. Jaco (ed.) *Patients, physicians and illness*. New York: Free Press

McMurdo, M.E. (2000) 'A healthy old age: realistic or futile goal?' *British Medical Journal*, Nov 2000, 321: 1149–51

Meddings, F. and Haith-Cooper, M. (2008) 'Culture and communication in ethical care'. *Nursing Ethics*, 15 (1): 52–60

Meredith, I.S., Orlando, M., Humphrey, N., Camp, P. and Sherbourne, C.D. (2001) 'Are better ratings of the patient-provider relationship associated with higher quality of care for depression?' *Medical Care*, 39: 349–60

Mezirow, J. (1981) 'A critical theory of adult learning and adult education'. *Adult Education*, 32: 3–24

Miller, P. and Eisenburg, N. (1988) in Omdahl, B. and O'Donnel, C. (1999) 'Emotional, contagion, empathetic concern and communicative responsiveness as variables affecting nurses' stress and occupational commitment'. *Journal of Advanced Nursing*, 29 (6): 1351–9

Mitchell, P.H. (1973) *Concepts basic to nursing*. New York: McGraw-Hill

Moccia, P (1988) 'At the faultline: social activism and caring'. *Nursing Outlook*, 36(1): 30–3

Moon, J. (1999) *Learning journals: a handbook for academics, students and professional development*. London: Kogan Page

Moon, J. (2004) *A handbook of reflective and experiential learning: theory and practice*. London: Routledge

Moon, G. and Gillespie, R. (1995) *Society and health: an introduction to social science for health professionals*. London: Routledge

Morrison, P. (1991) 'The caring attitude in nursing practice: a repertory grid study of trained nurse perceptions'. *Nurse Education Today*, 11: 3–12

Morrison, P. (1992) *Caring and nursing: professional caring in nursing practice*. Aldershot: Avebury

Morse, J., Bottorff, J., O'Brien, B. and Solberg, S. (1992) 'Beyond empathy: expanding expressions of caring'. *Journal of Advanced Nursing*, 17: 809–21

Morse, J., Solberg, S., Neander, W. and Johnson, J. (1990) 'Concepts of caring and caring as a concept'. *Advances in Nursing Science*, 13: 1–14

Moullin, S. (2007) *Care in a new welfare society: unpaid care, welfare and employment*. London: IPPR

National Council for Palliative Care (2006) *Introductory guide to end of life care in care homes*. NHS End of Life Care Programme available at **www.endoflifecare.nhs.uk/eolc**

NHS Executive (1999) *Clinical governance: quality in the new NHS*. London: HMSO

NHS Information Centre (2007) The Drugs Bill. **www.ic.nhs.uk**

NHS Management Executive (2003) *NHS chaplaincy: meeting the religious and spiritual needs of patients and staff*. London: HMSO

National Institute for Health and Clinical Excellence (2006) PH1 *Brief interventions and referral for smoking cessation: guidance*. London: HMSO

Nettleton, S. (2006) *Sociology of health and illness.* (2nd ed.). Cambridge: Polity Press

Nightingale, F. (1859) in Fagerström, L., Eriksson, K. and Bergbom Endberg, I. (1998) 'The patient's caring needs as a message of suffering'. *Journal of Advanced Nursing,* 28 (5): 978–87

Noddings, N. (1984) in Stockdale, M. and Warelow, P. (2000) 'Is complexity of care a paradox?' *Journal of Advanced Nursing,* 31(5): 1258–64

Nursing and Midwifery Council (NMC) (2004) *Standards of proficiency for pre-registration nursing education.* London: HMSO

Nursing and Midwifery Council (2007) *Essential skills clusters.* London: HMSO

Nursing and Midwifery Council (2008) *The code: standards for conduct, performance and ethics for nurses and midwives.* London: HMSO

Office for National Statistics (1999) *Health statistics quarterly* 2. London: HMSO

Office for National Statistics (2001) *Psychiatric morbidity report.* London: HMSO

Office for National Statistics (2003) *Better or worse: a longitudinal study of the mental health of adults in Great Britain.* London: HMSO

Omdahl, B. and O'Donnel, C. (1999) 'Emotional contagion, empathetic concern and communicative responsiveness as variables affecting nurses' stress and occupational commitment'. *Journal of Advanced Nursing,* 29 (6): 1351–9

Orem, D. (1980) *Nursing concepts of practice* (2nd ed.). New York: McGraw-Hill

Oulton, J.A. (1997) 'Inside view: let us show our capacity to care'. *International Nursing Review,* 44(5): 126

Ousey, K. and Johnson, M. (2007) 'Being a real nurse: concepts of caring in the clinical areas'. *Nurse Education in Practice,* 7: 150–5

Parsons (1981) in Benner, P. and Wrubel, J. (1989) *The primacy of caring.* New York: Addison Wesley

Pascall, G. (1997) *Social policy: a new feminist analysis.* London: Routledge

Peacock, J. and Nolan, P.N. (2000) 'Care under threat in the modern world'. *Journal of Advanced Nursing,* 32(5): 1066–70

Pepin, J. (1992) 'Family caring and caring in nursing'. *Journal of Nursing Scholarship,* 24(2): 127–31

Peplau, H.E. (1952) *Interpersonal relations in nursing.* New York: Putnam

Peplau, H.E. (1988) *Interpersonal relations in nursing* (2nd ed.). London: Macmillan

Peterson, A. and Waddell, C. (eds) (1998) *Health matters: a sociology of illness, prevention and care.* Buckingham: Open University Press

Platzer, D., Balke, D. and Ashford, D. (2000) 'An evaluation of process and outcomes from learning through reflective practice groups on a post-registration nursing course'. *Journal of Advanced Nursing,* 31: 689–95

Porter, S. and Ryan, S. (1996) 'Breaking the boundaries between nursing and sociology: a critical realist ethnography of the theory practice gap'. *Journal of Advanced Nursing,* 24(2): 413–20

Pryds-Jensen, K., Back-Pettersson, S. and Segesten K. (1993) 'The caring moment and the green thumb phenomenon among Swedish nurses'. *Nursing Science Quarterly,* 6(2): 98–104

Randle, J. (2001) 'Past caring? The influence of technology'. *Nurse Education in Practice,* 1: 157–65

Rich, A. and Parker, D.L. (1995) 'Reflection and critical incident analysis: ethical and moral implications of their use in nursing and midwifery education'. *Journal of Advanced Nursing*, 22: 1050–7

Riches, G. and Dawson, P. (2000) *An intimate loneliness*. Buckingham: Open University Press

Rideout, E. (ed.) (2001) *Transforming nursing education through problem based learning*. London: Jones and Bartlett

Roach, S. (1984) *Caring: the human mode of being*. Toronto: University of Toronto

Rogers, C.R. (1967) *On becoming a person: a therapist's view of psychotherapy*. London: Constable

Roper, N., Logan, W. and Tierney, A .(2000) *The Roper–Logan–Tierney model of nursing based on activities of living*. Edinburgh: Churchill Livingstone

Ross, L. (1995) 'The spiritual dimension'. *International Journal of Nursing Studies*, 32: 457–68

Routasalo, P. (1999) 'Physical touch in nursing studies: a literature review'. *Journal of Advanced Nursing*, 30(4): 843–50

Roy, C. (1980) 'The Roy adaptation model', in Riehl, J.P. and Roy, C. (eds) *Conceptual models for nursing practice*. New York: Appleton-Century-Crofts

Rush, B. and Cook, J. (2006) 'What makes a good nurse? Views of patients and carers'. *British Journal of Nursing*, 15 (7): 382–5

Russel, P. (2007) in Hogston, R. and Marjoram, B.A. (2007) *Foundations of nursing practice: leading the way*. Basingstoke: Palgrave Macmillan

Ryan Belcher, J.R. and Brittain Fish, L.J. (1990) 'Hildegard E. Peplau', in George, J.B. (ed.) *Nursing theories: the base for professional nursing practice* (3rd ed.). California: Prentice Hall

SAGA (2007) *Healthy living: complementary therapies. Therapies most likely to make it into mainstream treatment.* **www.saga.co.uk/health/healthyliving/complementarytherapies**

Saks, M. (1994) 'Alternative medicine', in Gabe, J., Kelleher, D. and Williams, G. (eds) *Challenging medicine*. London: Routledge

Salvage, J. (2001) 'New year revolution'. *Nursing Times*, 97(1): 21

Sandell R., Lazaar, A., Grant, J., Carlsson, Shubert, J. and Broberg, J. (2007) 'Therapist attitudes and patient outcomes'. *Psychotherapy Research*, March, 17 (2): 196–204

Sarkis, J. and Skoner, M. (1987) 'An analysis of the concept of holism in nursing literature'. *Holistic Nursing Practice*, 2(1): 61–9

Schön, D. (1983) *How professionals think in action*. New York: Basic Books

Scottish Executive, NHS (2006) *Delivering care, enabling health: Harnessing the nursing, midwifery and allied health professions' contribution to implementing Delivering for Health in Scotland*. Edinburgh: Scottish Executive

Seale, C. (1998) *Constructing death*. Cambridge: Cambridge University Press

Secretary of State for Health (1998) *A first class service*. London: The Stationery Office

Shannon, C. and Weaver, W. (1949) *The mathematical theory of communication*. Urbana: University of Illinois Press

Shiber, S. and Larson, E. (1991) 'Evaluating the quality of caring: structures, process and outcome'. *Holistic Nursing Practice*, 5: 57–66

Shumay, D., Maskarineo, G., Kakai, H. and Gotay, C. (2001) 'Why some cancer patients choose complementary and alternative medicine instead of conventional treatment'. *The Journal of Family Practice*, December, 50: 1067

Sitzer, V.A. (1996) in Clochsy, J., Brue, C., Cardin, S., Whittaker, A. and Rudy, E. (eds) *Critical care nursing* (2nd ed.). Philadelphia: Saunders

Skegg, P. (1984) *Law, ethics and medicine*. Oxford: Clarendon Press

Smith, P. (1992) *The emotional labour of nursing*. Basingstoke: Macmillan

Smith, F.B. (1982) *Florence Nightingale, reputation and power*. London: Croom Helm

Social Care Institute for Excellence (2004) *Briefing paper: terminal care in care homes*. London: SCIE

Social Care Institute for Excellence (2006) *Practice Guide 9. Dignity in Care*. November. London: SCIE

Sourial, S. (1997) 'An analysis of caring'. *Journal of Advanced Nursing*, 26: 1189–92

Stickley, T. (2002) 'Counselling and mental health nursing: a qualitative study'. *Journal of Psychiatric and Mental Health Nursing*, 9: 301–8

Stockdale, M. and Warelow, P. (2000) 'Is complexity of care a paradox?' *Journal of Advanced Nursing*, 31(5): 1258–64

Sturdy, D. (2008) 'Dependence and dignity'. *Nursing Older People*, 20 (3): 10

Sudnow, D. (1976) *Passing on: the social organisation of dying*. Englewood Cliffs, NJ: Prentice Hall

Swanson, K.M. (1993) 'Empirical development of a middle range theory of caring'. *Nursing Research*, 40: 161–6

Talerico, K.M. (2003) 'Person centred care: an important approach for 21st century health care'. *Journal of Psychosocial Nursing and Mental Health Services*, 41(11): 12–16

Tanner, C.A., Benner, P., Chesla, C. and Gordon, D. (1993) 'The phenomenology of knowing the patient'. *IMAGE: Journal of Nursing Scholarship*, 25(4): 273–80

Tanner, D. and Harris, J. (2008) *Working with older people*. London: Routledge in association with Community Care

Taylor, B. (2000) *Reflective practice: a guide for nurses and midwives*. Buckingham: Open University Press

Thomas, B., Hardy, S. and Cutting, P. (1996) *Stuart and Sundeen's mental health practice*. London: Mosby

Thompson, N. (2003) *Promoting equality* (2nd ed.). London: Macmillan

Travelbee, J. (1971) *Interpersonal aspects of mursing* (2nd ed.). Philadelphia: F.A. Davis

Turner, B. (1995) *Medical power and social knowledge* (2nd ed.). London: Sage

Turner, L. (1997) 'Euthanasia and distinctive horizons of moral reasoning'. *Mortality*, 2(3): 191–206

Tutton, E. (1991) 'Breaking the mould', in McMahon, R. and Pearson, A. (eds) *Nursing as therapy*. Suffolk: Chapman and Hall

United Kingdom Central Council for Nursing, Midwifery and Health Visiting (1999) *Fitness for practice*. London: UKCC

Valentine, K. (1989) 'Caring is more than kindness: modelling its complexities'. *Jona*, 19(11): 28–35

Warelow, P.J. (1996) 'Is caring the ethical ideal?' *Journal of Advanced Nursing*, 24(40): 655–61

Waters, A. (2008) 'Mind your differentials'. *Nursing Standard*, 22(18): 18–21

Watson, J. (1985) *Nursing: human science and human care: a theory of nursing*. New York: National League for Nursing Press

Webb, C. (1992) 'What is nursing?' *British Journal of Nursing*, 1(11): 567–8

Webber, P.B. (2002) 'A curriculum framework for nursing'. *Journal of Nursing Education*, 41(1): 15–25

White, J. (1995) 'Patterns of knowing: review, critique and update'. *Advances in Nursing Science*, 17(4): 73–86

Wilde Larsson, B. and Larsson, G. (1999) 'Patients' views on quality of care: do they merely reflect their sense of coherence?' *Journal of Advanced Nursing*, 30(1): 33–9

Wood, J. (2004) *Communication theories in action: an introduction*. Belmont: Wadsworth/Thomson Learning

Wooten, P. (1992) in McCreaddie and Wiggins (2008) op cit.

Young, A.P. (1994) *Law and professional conduct in nursing*. London: Scutari Press

WEBSITES

news.bbc.co.uk/1/hi/england/manchester/7118114.stm (accessed 28.1.08)

www.dh.gov.uk/en/Publicationsandstatistics/PublishedSurvey/Nationalsurvey ofNHSpatients/index.html

New Deal for Junior Doctors at www.dhsspsmi.gov.uk/scujunior doc-2

Index

Added to the page number, 'f' denotes a figure